YOUR HEART
KNOWS HOW TO
HEAL YOU

THE SACRED MEDICINE OF THE
FOUR CHAMBERS OF THE HEART

CISSI WILLIAMS

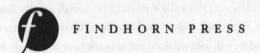

FINDHORN PRESS

Findhorn Press
One Park Street
Rochester, Vermont 05767
www.findhornpress.com

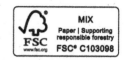

Findhorn Press is a division of Inner Traditions International

Disclaimer

The information in this book is given in good faith and is neither intended to diagnose any physical or mental condition nor to serve as a substitute for informed medical advice or care. Please contact your health professional for medical advice and treatment. Neither author nor publisher can be held liable by any person for any loss or damage whatsoever which may arise from the use of this book or any of the information therein.

Cataloging-in-Publication data for this title is available from the Library of Congress

ISBN 979-8-88850-204-4 (print)
ISBN 979-8-88850-205-1 (ebook)

Printed and bound in the United States by Lake Book Manufacturing, LLC

10 9 8 7 6 5 4 3 2 1

Edited by Susan Kemp
Illustrations by Damian Keenan (heart) and Alan Williams (heart chambers)
Design and layout by Damian Keenan
This book was typeset in Adobe Garamond Pro with ITC Century Std Book Condensed, and Museo used as display typefaces.

To send correspondence to the author of this book, mail a first-class letter to the author c/o Inner Traditions • Bear & Company, One Park Street, Rochester, VT 05767, USA and we will forward the communication, or contact the author directly at **https://www.cissiwilliams.com**.

For all the mothers and grandmothers,
sisters, and daughters—may we awaken the
feminine wisdom that is embedded within
our bones, flowing through our veins, and
wired into our DNA, so that we can weave her
healing medicine into our world.

Contents

Foreword
by HeatherAsh Amara

Imagine meeting a wise woman in the woods—or perhaps in the middle of New York City—your choice! She opens her cabin, or apartment, door and beckons you to enter. You feel completely safe and at ease. She invites you to sit down and, as you sink into a welcoming couch, she puts the kettle on to boil. As you look around you see herbs hanging from the rafters, notice jars of homemade tinctures, and salves on the shelves. A cat lazily stretches and is soon purring in your lap. With laughter in her eyes your host hands you a steaming mug of tea and sits facing you. You feel her stillness, the soothing gaze of her presence. You also feel the weight of her life experiences, her heart-break and heart-mend. You know you can trust her with your fears as well as your secrets.

"So, my dear," she says, "are you ready to heal your heart?"

Your heart leaps with a YES! And you know you are about to go on a very important inner journey.

I believe each of us is deeply craving such a wise elder to make us tea, hold our hand, and guide us through uncertain times back to our centre and faith.

Your Heart Knows How to Heal You is such a wise elder, lovingly handed to you with a cup of tea from the beautiful heart of Cissi Williams.

So often, instead of sitting in the presence of nurturing wisdom, we are trapped in busyness, distraction, and overwhelm. Instead of feeling our divinity, our worth gets tied into who we think we should be. We strive to be perfect, to prove we are worthy, to be accepted. And inside we feel empty, or exhausted.

We have been led away from our own inner knowing with the illusion of an outside "fix." Instead of trusting our own wisdom we try to prove we are good enough.

Instead of receiving and opening to the blessings all around us, we give our energy away and ignore the longing of our soul.

Cissi knows all about the longings of our soul, and learning how to receive blessings. As a shamanic teacher, and as a naturopath and osteopath, Cissi has guided thousands on their individual journeys toward healing. I was blessed to be introduced to Cissi through a mutual friend, and have been a witness to two major turning points in her life: the death of her mother and her own shamanic rebirth when she had a heart attack.

For some, losing a beloved parent and later having a heart attack might cause a closing down, a fearful response to loss and uncertainty. But Cissi is a warrior goddess, so she knew it was time to stop everything so she could deeply listen to the message her heart was bringing her. Her years of study and healing others gave her the strength and courage to take the most difficult path: into the depths of her own heart and soul.

Shamanism is a path of direct revelation, not a path of rules and regulations. Like our imaginary wise woman, Cissi invites us to her hearth and puts the kettle on. She doesn't tell us what to do, but rather guides us on an inner journey through the four chambers of our own heart. She shows us how to access our own wisdom through aligning back to the circle within and without: with the seasons and the biological rhythmic pumping of our blood.

In the first chamber of our heart we learn how to let go and shed our old identities, wounds, and fears like autumn leaves. In the second chamber of our heart we embrace the darkness of winter and enter the womb-space of our own transformation. In the third chamber of our heart we turn towards the light of new beginnings and opening to receive the blessings of spring. And in the fourth chamber we fully embrace the light of our rebirth and share it into the world, ripe and abundant as summer fruit.

What is so remarkable about this book is its multiple layers of invitation to meet the Dark and Light Goddesses and integrate their wisdom. Cissi introduces us to the potent medicine of Dark Mother who represents the primordial darkness that births new life. Once we have met and embodied the Dark Goddesses, she introduces us to the Light Goddesses. The Light Goddesses medicine is nourishment so you can bloom and expand. Again, Cissi doesn't tell, just introduces us to the Dark and Light Goddesses; she guides us through shamanic journeys to personally meet of these energies and listen directly to their wisdom. These guided shamanic journeys are written out in the book, and also available in beautifully produced audio recordings that supplement the writings.

This mythic map of transformation will guide you to discover your own soul gifts, healing medicine, feminine power, and ancient magic. You will be awakened to see through the eye of the heart, and become the Wise Woman that you already are.

Cissi, thank you for guiding us to heal our hearts and re-awaken our connection to the goddess within.

—**HeatherAsh Amara**, author of *Warrior Goddess Training, The Warrior Heart Practice*, and *Wild, Willing, and Wise*

13

A Note from the Author

· · · · · ·

The information, techniques, tools and processes in this book, and any shamanic journeys shared in this book (and in audio format) are not intended to diagnose, treat, cure, or prevent any condition or disease, and it does not replace a diagnosis from a medical doctor or other healthcare professional.

This book explores a variety of alternative ways that can result in healing and are based on the author's personal experience and opinion, but these are for inspirational and informational purposes only, and are not intended to replace advice, or ongoing treatment, from your own doctor or other healthcare professional.

It is suggested the reader approach these shamanic journeys and healing processes with caution, as any journey into the psyche can bring up emotions and memories.

This book, and the shamanic journeys outlined in the book (and available as audio versions on cissiwilliams.com/heart), are not recommended for those with fragile mental states, or with diagnosed medical illnesses such as psychosis, schizophrenia, bipolar disorders, clinical depression, and acute anxiety.

Please seek advice from your doctor or healthcare professional for any concerns regarding your health and wellbeing, prior to taking advice from this book, as well as if any health concerns arise during the reading of this book (as well as afterwards).

Anyone who chooses to do the work outlined in this book, and do the shamanic journeys, must take full responsibility for their own wellbeing and experience.

Introduction

Your Vision Will Become Clear
Only When You Look into Your Heart.
Who Looks Outside, Dreams.
Who Looks Inside, Awakens.

— CARL JUNG

Can you sense an untapped potential within you, longing to be expressed? Yet, however much you try to access it, something seems to be in the way? Or maybe you are longing for inner peace, but your inner voice keeps talking to you about everything that's wrong with your life, with others, with the world, with you. The more you listen to this inner dialogue, the more stressed you feel. You just want this critical voice to be quiet, so you can get some peace, but it chatters endlessly.

Or perhaps you feel trapped in a whirlwind of emotions—such as bitterness, blame, overwhelm, anxiety, or inner turmoil—and your mind keeps raging at others for events that took place in the past. You want to feel happy again, but it is as if you can't find the door that will lead you out of this dark place.

I've experienced all of this, and I want you to know that there is a way for you to heal this. My life today is so different from how it used to be. That inner voice that used to torment me from morning till night is quiet.

I'm no longer poisoned by inner wounds that had become infected and toxic, because I gained and utilized powerful tools to heal and transform those old wounds.

But most of all, I've tapped into an incredible source of feminine wisdom, like an ancient healing power more magical than I could have ever imagined.

All of this happened thanks to my heart finally making sure I listened to its whispers, and as I did, my heart healed me. Your heart can heal you too, if you are ready to listen to it.

Your heart is like a wise teacher who knows your highest potential and wants you to awaken this within you. To help you reach that potential, your heart may send you challenges as spiritual opportunities that invite you to go deeper on your healing journey. While the outside world might see these challenges as "bad," they may be exactly what is needed for you to become all that you are meant to be.

Stars cannot shine without the darkness of the night

Just as stars cannot shine without the darkness of the night, a diamond cannot be formed without pressure being exerted upon it.

You are meant to develop your inner diamond so that you can share your light and unique gifts with others. And for your inner diamond to form, you may need the pressure of various challenges coming into your life. These can often be experienced as periods of intense darkness.

Unfortunately, no one really teaches us how to move through these dark periods of our lives, so we often end up feeling that we have "failed" or something is "wrong" with us.

The self-help community says, "just change your thoughts," and the pharmaceutical industry says, "we have a pill for that." And often our loved ones freak out when they see us low and lacking in enthusiasm.

How do we deal with it ourselves? Usually by trying to avoid the feelings as much as possible, so we escape into our heads by distracting ourselves with work, watching TV, eating, drinking, focusing on everything else, all so that we don't have to deal with the real underlying issue that needs our attention.

But why do we go through these periods of intense darkness? Is something wrong with us when we experience this? Or is it perhaps a metaphor for how the night is always the darkest just before dawn breaks?

For many of us, this darkness is like an invitation from our soul, urging us to go *deeper* on our healing journey—so instead of avoiding this darkness, we are being invited to journey *into* it. These invitations tend to show up through different hardships, such as an illness, the loss of a relationship, or the ending of an aspect of our lives.

Initially, we may feel confused and overwhelmed by this challenge, but when we start to view what is happening as an invitation from our soul, then we come to understand that this upheaval is actually a doorway into a sacred, healing journey.

Trust that whatever challenge you've experienced in your life, whatever turmoil you've been going through, whichever path you've been on, has all led you here—to this place of even deeper healing—a healing that will develop your inner diamond even more, so it can shine and glisten like a star in the night.

You've already begun

Notice how much wisdom you have already awakened within you from the experiences you've been through. Consider one previous challenge you've had and overcome, and notice what it taught you. Witness the wisdom you gained.

Can you see how that challenge made you the person you are today? How that particular hardship shifted your perception so much that you were able to let go of old identities that no longer served you and move through your own rebirth, where you expanded into a new expression of your unique self.

This is the sacred medicine these challenges brought to you, and we have all experienced them.

Therefore, trust that you already know how to heal and connect with your inner wisdom, as you have done it many times already in your life. And through this book, your heart will guide you even *deeper*, taking you on an incredible journey of healing, transformation, magic, and rebirth. Just like mine did for me.

But before we start our healing journey together, let me tell you a story of how some of these challenges helped me to heal. This story will take us all the way back to a cold winter day in Stockholm, Sweden, in 1967.

Dancing between the light and the dark

On a full moon, just before midday a few days before the winter solstice, I was born in a hospital in Stockholm. I entered this world during the darkest month, but with the light from the moon and the sun brightening up my arrival.

My mum was the light of my life, while my dad brought in the darkness. He had been a young man, filled with an exuberant zest for life, until he crashed his car into a mountain wall when he was 24. The back of his skull was squashed into his brain, and one vertebra in his lower back got crushed, leaving him initially paralysed—and a few centimetres shorter. He was in a coma for eight days, and the doctors told my mum that if he were to ever wake up, he would be different.

My dad did wake up, and he was different, as he could no longer control his temper. He spent the next six months teaching himself how to walk again. During that time, his friends would come over every weekend with a deck of cards and vodka to cheer him up. By the time I was born a few years later, he was an alcoholic.

I never knew my dad the way he had been before the accident. I only knew him as the man imprisoned by the vodka demon. I could see how tormented he was, like a wounded animal lashing out for the slightest thing. He was a very sensitive man, with a big heart and a deep love of nature, but it was as if the darkness in him ate more and more of his life force, with each passing year.

As I child I was often told that I was like my dad, the way he was before the accident. I don't know if that had anything to do with it, but for some reason, a lot of his anger was directed at me. I constantly felt as if I was walking around on eggshells, expecting an outburst at any moment. I became an expert in reading his energy so that I could quickly figure out if it was safe to be in the same room as him.

When I was around 12, I started to realize that something wasn't quite right at home. I was at my best friend's apartment, and her family invited me to stay for dinner. Mealtimes always made me anxious, as Dad's temper could explode while we were eating. Once we were eating salted fried herring (it is as horrid as it sounds) and I had to swallow it down with milk in order not to vomit. Dad saw this and exploded. He reached over the table, grabbed me by my hair, and threw me into the wall.

Therefore, I was quite anxious as I sat down for a meal with my friend's family. I kept looking at her dad, waiting for him to lash out—but he didn't. Instead, he spoke softly, smiled, and chatted lovingly with his family. I was stunned. This was a new experience for me.

That was the moment I realized my dad's behaviour wasn't normal. As I started to rebel against what was happening at home, I got the blame for upsetting Dad. My Mum tried to make me see that if only I could be nicer to Dad, and not anger him so much, then everything would be fine. But I couldn't stop rebelling. It was as if there was a fire in me, roaring, and I had to give voice to it. Doing so only made it more tense at home.

Fortunately, it turned out that I was very good academically. Both my parents had to finish school early—around the age of 13—and my dad was proud of my academic achievements. This meant that whenever I sat at the dining table with a schoolbook open, he never lashed out at me. Studying became my safety zone.

Despite this, I felt I was trapped in a nightmare, a bad dream that never seemed to end. I was very lucky though, because Mum did the best she could and made sure we had two homes—a flat where my sister and I lived with her during the week, and a summer house where we all lived together with Dad during the weekends and on school holidays. This meant that the difficult experience I had at home was only part-time, which again provided the contrast of darkness and light. Life with Mum was easy, happy, and light-filled, while life with Dad was stressful, challenging, and filled with a heavy darkness.

When I was 18, I set off travelling. I can now see how this was an attempt on my part to escape the chaos at home. I didn't know that I would leave Sweden but keep on carrying those deep inner wounds with me. And these wounds eventually demanded to be healed.

Hearing the voice of spirit

A year or so into my travels, I met an astrologer in Varanasi, India, who told me I was very depressed and disconnected from life. I could not relate at all to what he was talking about, as I felt quite happy. A bit empty perhaps, as if I lived in a void, but at least I didn't walk around on eggshells anymore.

Now in hindsight I can see how frozen I was, as if I just lived from my head, planning on where to go next, just drifting from place to place, avoiding setting down roots anywhere. As I had felt so trapped at home, I now *craved* freedom.

Then, a few more years into my travelling, when I was living in Tokyo in my early 20s, I met someone. I remember being in the kitchen, with a cup of tea in my hand, when this man from London, a decade my senior, came up to me. I had this inner voice telling me, "Stay away from him," which I thought was a bit odd. I ignored the warning, and we ended up together.

Our relationship opened the gates to all my inner wounds and within a short space of time I abandoned my former self. I was victim-oriented, controlling, needy, and had a deep-seated fear of being rejected. I also developed an eating disorder to try to numb my inner turmoil. I would binge eat and then purge, and it would exhaust me so much, I would fall asleep afterwards.

Hardly surprisingly, this relationship ended and, as it did, I fell into a deep depression, into a darkness that seemed to drain me of my life force. This was in the autumn of 1992. I was 24 years old and living alone in London. I remember having this thought that I looked like a shiny apple on the outside, but inside I was completely rotten.

Then one night, in my tiny little room on Pond Street in Hampstead, I had a dream where I saw myself hanging dead from the ceiling. As I woke up, covered in sweat, I knew I had to change. I could no longer keep blaming my dad, or my ex-boyfriend, for how I was feeling. I knew I had to change my thoughts, but I had no idea how to. The nightmare of seeing myself hanging from the ceiling had really shaken me, as if it was giving me a glimpse into my future, so I sat up in bed, pulled the duvet tighter around me, and I prayed. I had never prayed before, but I was desperate. I didn't know who else to turn to, so I turned to the Universe, hoping to get an answer.

Nothing seemed to happen at first, but then I got this inner feeling that I should go back to Stockholm. I immediately booked a flight back home.

The very next day I found myself in a spiritual bookshop in my hometown, where three books seemed to just land in my lap—*The Power Is Within You* by Louise Hay, *Love Is the Answer* by Gerald Jampolsky, and *Creative Visualization* by Shakti Gawain.

As I started reading these books, I could feel myself getting lighter. It was as if a door to another universe had opened, a light-filled universe, that led me out from this dark world I previously felt trapped in.

I realized that my prayer had been answered as these books gave me the tools I needed to help me change my thinking and connect with the light from Spirit—a light I recognized was also in me. This was such a huge revelation for me; that this light existed within me!

As I kept focusing on this inner light, as I kept choosing love instead of fear, the darkness began to recede. Within six weeks my depression was gone, and within four months my bulimic behaviours had stopped. Just from me *choosing* to focus on the light, *choosing* to focus on love, *choosing* to heal my thinking.

Through healing my thoughts, my mind became more peaceful, which allowed me to hear Spirit's Voice more clearly. The inner critical voice—the ego's voice—is so loud and noisy, while Spirit's Voice is soft, gentle, and loving, so we can only hear it when our mind is peaceful. This loving inner voice guided me to study osteopathy and naturopathy. So one year after having reached rock-bottom, I found myself enrolled in a four-year university degree in Osteopathic Medicine in London.

This loving inner voice also guided me to meet my husband! As I was in my fourth year of osteopathy training, a new clinic tutor walked in, Mr. Williams, and the moment I saw him I heard this inner voice say: "That's your husband!" We were married on the full moon at the summer solstice the following year, and we are still going strong, nearly three decades later.

I started to trust this inner, loving voice, and it guided me to later study hypnosis, neuro-linguistic programming, and various shamanic healing modalities (including those from the Incas, Norse, and Celts).

I was passionate about sharing with others what I knew—that we have this amazing power within us to heal. Over the next two decades, I helped thousands of clients, patients, and students tune into their inner wisdom. I also set up two spiritual wellbeing magazines—one in Sweden and one in the UK—and founded the podcast *Awaken Your Inner Wisdom*.

I had no idea that I was about to receive an invitation from my heart to step through another door of initiation that would lead me into the magical realm of the ancient wisdom found in the feminine.

A message from my heart

On a full moon in November, just a few weeks shy of my 52nd birthday—what is it with me and full moons?—I was sitting on my sofa with my laptop, working on an episode for my podcast, when I suddenly experienced extreme chest pain. It was so bad I fell to my knees. The pain was radiating up to my right jaw, and it was hard for me to breathe. The pain lasted for perhaps five to ten minutes. Then it eased, and I felt better.

I sent a text message to my husband, who was teaching osteopathy in London, where I wrote: "Don't worry, but I've just had extreme chest pain, radiating up to my right jaw, but I'm fine now."

Then I sat back down on the sofa and continued editing my podcast episode, as if nothing had happened.

My husband, on the other hand, freaked out and drove straight back home. He pleaded with me to see the GP, but I insisted I was fine now, and I absolutely had to finish this podcast episode, so seeing the GP had to wait.

Then the pain came back, although not as bad. I still felt it was no big deal, but to ease my husband's worry, I phoned the GP surgery and was told to come in immediately. I took an ECG test, which revealed signs of a heart attack. I was still ignoring the seriousness of what had happened, but the GP told me that if I felt worse, I needed to go to the hospital.

Over the next few days, I still had chest pain on and off. My husband was getting quite frustrated with me as I did not seem too concerned. In the end, he persuaded me to come with him to John Radcliffe Hospital in Oxford, so off we went. As we were sitting there in the waiting room, I took out my laptop from my bag and started typing away.

My husband looked at me and said, "There's something really wrong with this picture, with you sitting here at the ER with your laptop." I just smiled at him reassuringly and, as I felt fine, I kept on working. I was sure the wait would be a little while, and I just had a tiny bit left to finish off and then the podcast episode would be ready to be uploaded.

At that moment my name was called, and I went to have various blood tests and another ECG done. This too showed signs of a heart attack and my blood pressure was really high. They kept a cannula in my vein in my left arm to make it easier to give me any medication or take more blood. This proved to be very effective in stopping me from working on my laptop, as I could not bend my elbow.

I was taken to another waiting room, and by this stage we had been at the hospital for a few hours, so my husband went to get some sandwiches. This was the first time I was completely alone. And that is when it hit me, as I was sitting there, looking out through the windows at the grey November sky. I had had a heart attack! Just as my mum had when she was only 48.

My mind finally stopped being in denial and I registered the enormity of the situation. I felt overwhelmed by sadness and grief and fear, as I had seen what the heart attack did to Mum. She became a prisoner of her own body.

It suddenly dawned on me that I had two options. I could either go down one road, feeling helpless, thinking that this was just my fate, as it is in my genetics (we have a blood clotting disorder). I felt my inner fear tempt me down that path, as if an arm was reaching up from beneath me, trying to pull me down a dark tunnel of helplessness.

Or I could choose the other option, where I could see the heart attack as an invitation to awaken—a doorway into a deeper wisdom.

I decided to choose the second.

At that moment, in the waiting room at the hospital, as I made this decision to let my heart heal me, I was filled with a deep inner peace. I just knew that somehow everything would be fine.

A journey of rebirth

I had absolutely no idea the amazing journey my heart would take me on—a journey that would awaken an ancient feminine power within me that not only healed my body, but also healed *me*. It transformed *me*. It ignited the magic in *me*.

This journey took me through my own rebirth, where I started to fully embody the Wise Woman within my core—and, my goodness, she is fierce! She is like an ancient witch, full of wild magic, ancestral wisdom, and feminine power. She was always there, like an untapped potential, deep within my core and, although I could sense her, I could never fully connect with her. This is because I had tried to reach her with my head, and now I know she can only be reached through the heart.

It was my heart that was the doorway into everything I had previously longed for. As I listened to its whispers, it took me on an amazing shamanic journey into the medicine found in its four chambers—a medicine of healing, transformation, magic, and rebirth. A medicine that dances with the sacred darkness and the magical light, being fully in tune with the seasons of Mother Earth.

As I guide you through the chapters of this book, your heart will lead you on a shamanic journey of deep healing, awakening the Wise Woman within you. And trust me—she is AMAZING! She is FIERCE! She is MAGICAL! She is POWERFUL! She is the one that opens the door to all the untapped potential that is longing to be expressed through you.

Each chapter in this book is a doorway that leads into a deeper wisdom and magic for you, and every chapter ends with a shamanic journey where you discover the healing medicine and feminine power that is yours to claim. You can access the recordings of these shamanic journeys on **cissiwilliams.com/heart**.

The first part of the book helps you to move from your head to your heart and sets the foundation for the rest of the book, allowing you to open to the wisdom found in your heart. Your heart is the compass you follow on this sacred journey, guiding you as you travel into the World of Spirit with the Tree of Life as your map.

The second part of the book is when your shamanic journey begins. We venture into the four chambers of your heart, where you experience the sacred medicine each chamber holds for you. Here, you are invited to fully embrace your heart as your teacher, as it will guide you to the insights and learnings you need in order to heal and transform deeply.

The third part of the book helps you tune into the whispers from your heart, so you can weave your heart's loving energy into your world, filling your relationships, dreams, visions, and important life areas with all of the healing medicine, soul gifts, clarity, and wisdom that you have awakened within you by moving through each chapter in this book.

The material in this book is the culmination of my experience from guiding more than 25,000 healing sessions, teaching thousands of students, and helping many more connect with their inner wisdom.

Many of the shamanic journeys in this book were recorded live in the shamanic energy medicine practitioner training I run, so I know how powerful they are—not just from having done these shamanic journeys myself, but also from having guided my students on them.

As you let your heart guide you on this healing journey, and you give yourself time to listen to the shamanic journey at the end of each chapter, you will move through your own healing, transformation, and rebirth, awakening the Wise Woman within you. But before we set off on this magical journey together, let us first get to know who this Wise Woman is.

Who Is This Wise Woman?

Within every woman there lives a powerful force,
filled with good instincts, passionate creativity,
and ageless knowing.
She is the Wild Woman, who represents
the instinctual nature of women.
— CLARISSA PINKOLA ESTES

The Wise Woman is the ancient feminine wisdom wired into your DNA and maternal mitochondria, inherited through the mother line—your direct link with the Ancient Mother. She is the one who governs your wellbeing, and she responds to the natural elements of earth, water, air, and fire, and to the cycles of darkness and light.

She knows it's the darkness of the womb that births the light of new life. She also knows this new life must continue to receive light to grow, so she is always seeking the light and letting it nourish her.

In the old days, those who embodied this ancient feminine wisdom were called Wise Women, wise folks, the wise ones, folk healers, *völvas* (meaning staff carrier, who were female shamans in the Norse tradition), and cunning folks. Cunning comes from the Swedish word *kunnig*, which means knowledgeable.

Before Christianity took hold in Europe, these Wise Women were revered for their knowledge as healers, midwives, herbalists, mystics, oracles, and seers. As Christianity gained more power, the attitude changed. Instead of being revered, they became feared. The wise ones became "witches."

The older meaning for the word *witch* comes from the word *wicche*, which means wise one, and also from the word *wit*, which means wise, and to bind, shape, and alter. These Wise Women knew how to bind, shape, and alter reality, by changing the energetic hold of the past, and by *weaving* and *spinning* new energy into the future—through healing practices, songs, sacred ceremonies, binding spells, and shamanic journeying into the World of Spirit.

The church saw these Wise Women as a threat to their authority, as the Wise Ones were able to communicate directly with the Divine. To silence them, the Wise Women were made into "evil witches," and as the witch trials swept through Europe, this ancient feminine wisdom was pushed underground, as it was no longer safe to practice. This forced women to fear their own feminine power and magic.

Not only was our perception of the Wise Ones distorted, but the church also altered our view on the Divine Mothers of Darkness, the Dark Mothers. They did this by changing the stories around them. For example, the Norse dark goddess Hel had been worshipped as a beautiful and powerful Mother Goddess for thousands of years, before she was twisted into the miserable ruler of hell.

Her name, Hel, in Swedish means to heal (*hela*), whole (*hel*), sacred (*helig*), and hidden (*hölja*). Ancient pagans saw her as a sacred goddess who lived in a place of rebirth, where her divine fire was burning. She was able to heal the sick and give life to the dead so they could be reborn again. She represented the moon, where half of her was white, like the full moon, and half of her was dark blue, like the dark moon. In this older tradition, she was a life-giving and beautiful Dark Mother, seen as a portal that guides you into a new life.

But the church changed her into someone to be feared, as the ruler of hell. She was now portrayed as scary and miserable, where half of her was a skeleton woman, symbolising death, and the other half was a maiden, symbolising life. Distorting Hel's myth effectively stopped women from connecting with her. Women forgot that the Dark Mother Hel was also the bringer of life.

Who is the Dark Mother?

The Dark Mother is the primordial darkness from and through which all life stems. You were born from her sacred womb, from her loving heart. Your heartbeat is linked with her heartbeat, and with the heartbeat of all the women who have walked before you, and will come after you.

The Dark Mother is a lunar goddess of the night, and she has been vilified over centuries and made into something evil and scary.

But she's not. She is loving and fiercely compassionate, as she helps you to remove that which has blocked you from remembering your real feminine wisdom, power, and magic.

For thousands of years, she was worshipped as the Mother who gave birth to all life. The ancients knew, as evidenced in their mythologies, that the darkness births the light.

In Norse mythology, the goddess of the night is called Natt. She is the mother of Day and Earth. She is most likely also the mother of Mani (moon) and Sol (sun).

In Greek mythology the goddess of the night is called Nyx. She is the mother of Hemera (day) and Aether (brightness).

In Egyptian mythology, the goddess of the night is called Nut. She is the mother of Isis, who was seen as both a solar and a lunar goddess.

Just as the goddesses of ancient mythology birthed light from the dark, we do the same. We are starlight in a physical body, and our journey into this world begins in the darkness of the womb. We journey from darkness to light to darkness again and again in our personal mythos.

All these Dark Mothers represented the primordial darkness that births new life, including the Norse goddess Hel, the Celtic goddess Cerridwen, the Greek goddess Hecate, and the Black Madonna found in Christianity. You will meet them all in chapter four. These goddesses are all daughters of the primordial Dark Mother, with similar powers and medicines, expressed in their own unique ways, as if they speak the same language with different accents. Collectively, they invite you to step through the portal of transformation, where you move into the sacred darkness to be born into something new.

In Mother Earth's seasons, the Dark Mothers are present in the autumn and winter, where the old must be released to birth something new. And then, in the spring and summer, the Divine Mothers of Light, the Light Mothers (solar goddesses) take over, nourishing the seeds of new life to blossom and give fruit.

Who are the Light Mothers?

In the Norse, Arctic, and Celtic traditions, the sun was often seen as feminine, as she is the bringer of life after a dark and cold winter.

Some of the most important solar goddesses are the Celtic goddess Brigid (also known as Brighid, Brighde, or Brid), and the Norse goddesses Freya and Idun. You will meet the Light Mothers in chapter six. They are the Light Mothers returning the nourishing rays of the sun to the land after a long winter, igniting the magic of love so that life can blossom.

Through this dance of darkness and light, we can see how both are needed for life to expand.

The healing medicine of darkness and light

Your body receives the healing medicine of darkness and light through the pineal gland, a small gland in the middle of the skull and the remnant of your third eye.

When the pineal gland registers darkness, it produces melatonin, which helps to recharge your brain, boost your immune system, strengthen your heart, improve your memory, and open the gateway to your psychic power, the intuition of your third eye.

Your body heals itself during the night, and the aging process is slowed down. That means the medicine of darkness heals and rebirths you, just like the healing energies of the Dark Mothers.

When your pineal gland registers sunlight, it strengthens your bones, reduces inflammation in your body, and boosts your serotonin levels, which uplifts your mood and helps you to feel calm and focused. It also increases your melatonin production at night, boosting all the medicinal qualities of the dark too.

For more information about the medicine of darkness and light, visit Dr. Azra Bertrand's website: azrabertrand.com.

The medicine of light gives you a direct link with the healing energies of the Light Mothers who give you the nourishment you need to blossom and expand; while the medicine of darkness gives you a direct link with the healing energies of the Dark Mothers, helping to rebirth you.

So let us begin this magical journey of awakening now, by first tuning into the wisdom found in your mystical heart—a wisdom that is like a loving teacher who knows how to guide you on your healing journey, where you learn how to dance with the sacred darkness and the magical light, enabling you to release the old and blossom into something new.

Part 1

From the Head
to the Heart

Your Heart Is a Teacher

In a conflict between the heart and the brain,
follow your heart.
— SWAMI VIVEKANANDA

There is an ancient prophecy from the Andes and Amazonas about the Condor and the Eagle, which describes how, a long time ago, humanity was split into two paths—the path of the Eagle and the path of the Condor.

The path of the Eagle is the path of the mind, of the masculine, of the linear, rational, and structured way of thinking—qualities appreciated in our modern world.

The path of the Condor is the path of the heart, of the feminine, of the intuitive, wise and magical way of being—qualities revered in ancient wisdom traditions where living in harmony with Mother Earth was seen as essential.

This ancient prophecy describes how, beginning in the 1490s, a 500-year period would begin where the Eagle people's way of life would become so powerful that it starts to dominate the world to the point that it nearly causes the Condor people's way of life to become extinct. When this happens, Mother Earth will begin to express this imbalance through fires, storms, flooding, hurricanes, and drought.

The opportunity will then arise for the Eagle and Condor to learn to fly together in the same sky in harmony with each other. And through them flying together, a new consciousness will be born, where the mind and the heart, the masculine and the feminine, are in balance with each other. The Q'ero Inca shamans from the high Andes refer to this as *Pachacuti*, which means turning the world right again. And as this shift happens, a new time for the earth begins.

I feel that this is where we are right now, at a choice point of moving from our heads to our hearts. So, we let our heart become our teacher, guiding us to what we need to heal so that we can come into balance again with our heart and mind, with the masculine and the feminine, and in this way create a new world.

I started my healing journey with healing my mind, through connecting with the light of Spirit, changing my thought patterns, and learning to focus on the light. The miracles from this were that I could forgive my dad fully, create a loving home with my husband and our two daughters, and find my path of helping others tune into their inner wisdom through my work with patients, clients, and students.

And then I was invited to step through a door that would lead me from my head to my heart, and into a realm of ancient feminine magic. This was when my heart would become my teacher.

My heart as my teacher

As my husband drove us back home from the hospital, I placed a hand over my heart and silently said, "I'm willing to heal, I'm willing to be guided, so show me what I need to know, and I promise I will listen."

And my heart did show me, in ways that surprised me.

The moment we got home, I felt a strong inner guidance to change my diet. Suddenly I lost all interest in foods I had normally eaten, and craved berries and vegetables instead.

I started making my own smoothies with strawberries, blueberries, blackcurrants, cranberries, and blackberries (all natural blood thinners).

I felt a strong guidance to take high doses of garlic capsules (garlic thins the blood and boosts the immune system).

My body also showed me immediately when it did not like a particular food item. When I took a bite from a potato gratin, my stomach threw it up within seconds, as if it was poison. The message was clear from my body—no potatoes for me.

It was as if my body took over guiding me on what to eat and what to avoid.

I could no longer have bread, potatoes, cheese, dairy, pasta, or rice. Only berries and vegetables. For six weeks! Then, after some time, I was allowed halloumi cheese. But no more potatoes; I still can't eat them!

This drastic change in my diet helped to thin my blood, and it quickly brought down my blood pressure to a normal range.

From the moment I asked my heart to show me what I needed, I was guided to make changes that helped my body to recover more quickly. None of this guidance was from my head. It was all from my heart. As an osteopath and naturopath, I would rarely recommend patients to go on such an extreme diet, but my body absolutely craved this. I recognized this inner guidance from when I had been pregnant before, as my body had taken charge then too, guiding me on what I should and should not eat.

During my second pregnancy, I suddenly developed an intense craving for dark chocolate, which turned out to be because of an iron deficiency. My body had signalled this to me before a blood test confirmed it, by giving me this intense craving (dark chocolate is a rich source in iron). Therefore, I knew that when I suddenly had a craving for a certain food, this was my body's wisdom communicating with me what it wanted me to eat. This change in diet was the first basic step of healing that my heart guided me to take. The main healing, however, came when my heart started to take me on shamanic journeys into the medicine found in each of the four chambers of the heart.

How the Four Chambers of the Heart Mirror the Four Seasons

· · · · · ·

The morning after I got home from the hospital, I felt this inner guidance to take a shamanic journey into the four chambers of my heart.

Being an osteopath, I work with different tissue structures of the body, and being a shamanic practitioner, I can "track" (seeing with my inner vision) the different energetic domains of our emotions, mind, soul, and spirit.

What I discovered as I followed the flow of the blood—in how it journeys through the four chambers of the heart—astounded me. I realized that the medicine found in each of the four heart chambers was the same medicine found in each of the four seasons.

Let me share in more detail the medicine I found in the four heart chambers, as we follow the flow of the blood through the heart.

First chamber of the heart—the medicine of healing and letting go

I followed the flow of the blood into the first chamber, which deals with the deoxygenated blood (blood that is reduced in oxygen, compared to the blood leaving the lungs) returning to the heart from the body. The body is represented in the picture here as the Tree of Life.

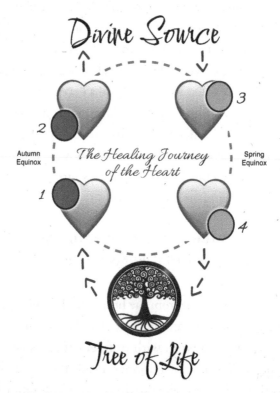

Figure 1: The body as the Tree of Life, the Divine Source as the lungs, and the four heart chambers.

I sensed how this deoxygenated blood represented that which was *poor in spirit* ("in-spiration," so lacking in "spirit"), or what we are meant to let go of so that we can *begin our healing journey* and later expand into something new.

This is like the medicine Mother Earth shows us in autumn, when she prepares to let go of the old (that which is "poor in spirit") so that new life can be born in the spring. Without this season's clearing and healing of the old, life can't expand the following year.

This is when we begin our journey that takes us through the portal of the autumn equinox into the sacred darkness of early winter.

Second chamber—the medicine of transformation

I then followed the flow of the blood into the second chamber of the heart, which is bigger than the first, as it prepares the blood to be pumped up to the lungs. I could sense here how this chamber deals with *transforming* that which we are meant to let go of and heal, preparing us to receive the light of something new.

This is similar to the medicine of early winter, when we are in the sacred darkness, transforming the old, preparing us for the arrival of new life as the light returns.

This is the season when we work with the Dark Mothers—you will meet them in chapter four—facing our shadows and inner wounds so that they can be transformed into light and wisdom.

Lungs as the Divine Source—receiving the light of new inspiration

As I followed the flow of the blood, I was taken to the lungs, where the blood goes to become oxygenated. I saw my lungs as a huge Cosmic Angel, *breathing in Spirit*, filling me with the light of new inspiration, visions, dreams, gifts, blessings, and nourishment. This Cosmic Angel was like the Divine Source, where the light-filled seeds of what's meant to be born already exist.

I could see how this too corresponded with the seasons of the year— this time the Winter Solstice when the light is being reborn in the darkness. This returning light contains the light-filled seeds of new life, hope, visions, and dreams. And the flow of the blood was showing me that what happens every year in nature also happens within my body with every heartbeat.

Third chamber—the medicine of the magical light

I then followed the flow of the blood into the third chamber of the heart, which deals with receiving all of the oxygen-rich blood from the lungs. I could sense how the medicine of this chamber was all about *receiving* the light from the heavens, as we need this light to nourish our new visions, dreams, and inspiration.

I could see how this chamber was like the season of early spring, when the light is returning to the land. This light nourishes the seeds of new life, as it's too early for them to be born yet. And as the seeds are nourished by the light from the heavens, the magic of creation happens! Life expands and blossoms.

Incidentally, this is where I had the problem in my heart, as I was too focused on giving all this light away to others, but not so good at receiving it for me.

Spring is the season when we work with the Light Mothers to ignite our inner magic, by being willing to receive their nourishing light. They then guide us through the portal of the spring equinox into the magical light of early summer.

Fourth chamber—the medicine of rebirth

I then followed the flow of the blood into the fourth chamber of the heart. This is the chamber that pumps all the oxygen-rich blood out into the whole body, so that it can be nourished and filled with life, the body being a metaphor for the world. I realized that the medicine of the fourth chamber was to help us to receive so much light that we move through our own rebirth. And as we are reborn, we can go into the world, sharing our gifts, inspiration, visions, and dreams with others—just as the fourth chamber shares all the oxygen-rich blood with the body.

This is what Mother Earth does in early summer, when she has moved through her own rebirth, allowing life to expand and blossom, so she can share her gifts with the world.

As you can see, this journey into the chambers of my heart awakened me into a deeper understanding of how we are meant to dance with the seasons of darkness and light of the feminine. This set me off on a shamanic journey of healing the deep wounds held within the feminine. As this wound healed, the Wise Woman within me awakened. As she will in you too.

I will soon take you on a shamanic journey in which you'll experience the medicine that each chamber of your heart holds for you. But before we go on this journey, let us first look at what shamanism is, and then also go through some guidelines for how to use the shamanic journeys, so you can benefit the most from their healing and transformational power.

What Is Shamanism?

If you have ever felt more alive while walking through a forest, more refreshed when swimming in the sea, or more connected while talking under the stars over a campfire, you have experienced one of the planet's oldest spiritual traditions.

Shamanism is the oldest known spiritual practice in the world, predating all religions. Some sources say it is more than 10,000 years old, others suggest it is more than 45,000 years old.

Shamanism has evolved in a variety of ways in different parts of the world, but these divergent threads share many similarities, such as the belief that everything is alive and has a spirit, and that we are all connected with all of life.

The actual word *shaman* seems to stem from the Tungus tribe in Siberia, meaning "one who knows," but those who serve as the shaman for their people were called different things depending on their culture. In the Sami culture—native people from the north of Sweden, Norway, Finland, and Russia—they are called *noaidis*, in the Norse tradition they were usually women called *völvas*, and the Peruvian Q'ero shamans are called *paqos*. These shamanic practitioners all work as intermediaries between the spirit world and our physical world, by being able to "track" (see, feel, hear, and know intuitively, through their body and inner vision) what is happening in the energetic domains of the emotions, mind, soul, and spirit.

Honouring the birth of the light in the darkness

Many of the ancient shamanic wisdom traditions honoured the passage of time by following the movement of the sun so that they could live in sync with the eternal changes of the seasons of darkness and light.

One such honoured moment was the birth of the light in the middle of the darkness, which takes place at the winter solstice—the darkest time of the year when the light returns.

This may have been one of the reasons they built sacred stone altars, such as Stonehenge in England, Machu Picchu in Peru, and Newgrange in Ireland, which are monuments perfectly aligned with the movement of the sun.

Stonehenge, located on the Salisbury plains in England, dates back roughly 4,500 years. The stones at Stonehenge are shaped and set up in such a way that they frame at least two of the most important events in the annual solar cycle: the midwinter sunset at the winter solstice; and the midsummer sunrise at the summer solstice.

Machu Picchu, located in the Andes mountains of Peru, was built in A.D. 1450 at the height of the Inca Empire. These ancient ruins were designed such that at the moment of dawn on the winter solstice, when the very first light rises over the distant mountains, the sun's light shines through one of the two windows of the Temple of the Sun and illuminates the ceremonial stone within.

Newgrange in Ireland is more than 5,000 years old, which pre-dates the Egyptian pyramids. It is an ancient earth temple, a passage tomb, where the first rays of the sun's golden light on winter solstice travel through it to light up the dark chamber within.

Tree of Life

Another common thread found in most ancient shamanic wisdom traditions is reference to the Tree of Life, which often symbolizes the following:

- The roots of the tree symbolize your connection with the earth, with the lower world, which is your unconscious mind and your past, connecting you with your ancestors.

- The branches symbolize your connection with the heavens, with the upper world, which is your higher consciousness, and that which you are becoming.

- The trunk symbolizes your connection with the middle world, which is your life here on Earth, the one you are consciously aware of.

- The west direction of the tree symbolizes the dying sun, that which is falling away. It represents the sacred darkness of the night, so it is linked with the Dark Mothers (lunar goddesses).

- The east direction of the tree symbolizes the rising sun, that which is being reborn—just as the sun is reborn every morning, after having "died" the previous night. It represents the magical light of morning and is therefore linked with the Light Mothers (solar goddesses).

- The Tree of Life symbolizes the eternal cycle of life—through its changing seasons—representing transformation and rebirth.

- Through its fruits it gives everlasting life, wisdom, and knowledge. These fruits—often apples—are a symbol of divine feminine wisdom that can only be gained through moving with the seasonal cycles of darkness and light.

The Tree of Life acts as a portal into the lower world, upper world, and middle world, so it gives us a map that we can follow when we do shamanic journeys, so that we can journey down into our roots, to the lower world to heal old wounds, and journey up to the upper world to receive new visions and dreams.

Seeing through the eye of the heart

A shamanic practitioner uses the eye of the heart to witness what her physical eyes cannot see, as the heart is the portal that connects us with the realm of our soul and spirit.

Black Elk was a medicine man and holy man of the Oglala Lakota (Sioux). He described how there is a space within the centre of the heart, where Great Spirit resides. This space is the eye of the heart, the eye that can receive visions to help others.

In *The Gospel of Mary* (written around the second century) Mary Magdalene asks Christ if a person who sees a vision sees it with the soul or with the spirit. Christ answers that a person does not see with the soul or with the spirit, rather with the "mind," which exists between these two.

Scholar of the divine feminine, Meggan Watterson, in her book *Mary Magdalene Revealed*, shares how the original word for "mind" in ancient Greek was the word *nous*, which means the "spiritual eye of the heart." So it is only through the "spiritual eye of the heart" that Mary Magdalene can have this vision of Christ, and she must learn to trust what she is seeing, without getting any outside validation.

It is the same when we do shamanic journeys. We must learn to trust our "spiritual eye of the heart"—so that we learn to trust our inner vision, our inner knowing, our inner feeling of what is taking place in the journey—and let go of our need for external validation.

You will develop your "eye of the heart" through the shamanic journeys found at the end of each chapter in this book.

Guidelines for Using the Shamanic Journeys in This Book

• • • • • •

All of the shamanic journeys in this book—for which you can find audio recordings at **cissiwilliams.com/heart**—start with us tuning into the light that shines in our mystical heart, as this light is the portal into the World of Spirit. This light is the "eye of the heart."

Letting go of the mind's need to understand

In the beginning, when we do shamanic journeys, the mind tries to interfere constantly, doubting everything we see, feel and experience. But the more we practice shamanic journeying, the more we start to trust the eye in our heart. It is like a trust muscle we develop the more that we practice.

Your heart becomes your shamanic guide

All of the shamanic journeys in this book are based on inner journeys I have taken myself. Through these journeys, I've guided many clients and students. The journeys are incredibly healing and transformational and are quite similar in their format to a shamanic healing session. Therefore, approach them as you would a healing session—the shaman is your own heart's wisdom guiding you on this journey. And instead of a shamanic practitioner "tracking" (seeing and sensing with their inner vision) what is happening in the journey, you are tracking through the eye of your heart.

Staying awake

I would recommend that you do the journeys sitting up and when you are feeling rested. This helps you have the energy you need to stay awake. If you notice that you often fall asleep in journeys, chances are you are also falling asleep to aspects of your life, so make sure you stay awake.

Sometimes you may find that you nod off during a particular part of the journey. Noticing when you nod off will give you a clue to what you are avoiding. This often happens when we avoid witnessing something that we are meant to heal or transform, or when we avoid receiving the healing medicine.

Everything you experience in the journey gives you clues to what is going on in your inner world, which also gives you insights to what is going on in your outer world. If you have problems acknowledging what needs to be healed and transformed, then chances are you fear journeying into the darkness. Perhaps because you fear what you will witness, and perhaps also because you fear the darkness.

If you notice this in yourself, then trust that the darkness *heals and rebirths you*. It is in the darkness of the night that the body heals. It is in the darkness of the womb that new life is formed. It is the darkness that births the light.

If you notice that you have problems receiving the healing medicine, then chances are that you fear receiving the nurturing light. Perhaps this is because you fear receiving light-filled support from the feminine, or maybe you feel unworthy of receiving.

Whatever the reason, if you notice that you block yourself from receiving the light, then know that without the light, nothing can grow. Therefore, if you want to expand and blossom in your life, then you must learn to receive this light, just as a flower opens to receive the healing medicine from the golden rays of the sun.

This book will help you to heal your relationship with both the darkness and the light of the feminine, so that you can embrace the medicine of both.

Being embodied during the shamanic journey

When you take shamanic journeys, it is helpful to use your breath and your body when you are releasing energies, so that you help to free yourself from the energetic hold of the past, enabling you to expand into something new.

In the journey, feel how you breathe out that which you no longer need, and use your hands to remove all heavy energy you want to release from your energy field. You can imagine you are handing it over to Mother Earth so that she can transform it into light.

Listen to my voice guiding you through the journeys

All of the shamanic journeys in this book are very powerful, and if you follow my voice as I guide you through them, and you use your breath and willingness to heal, then you will go much deeper when you journey. You access them on **cissiwilliams.com/heart**. Make sure that you can be completely undisturbed throughout the journey.

No note-taking during journeys

Never take notes during the shamanic journeys, as that will stop you from going deep, as your mind interferes with the journey. Instead, move from your head into your heart, and let your heart be your shamanic guide throughout the journey.

Then, once the journey has finished, you can engage your mind by writing down your insights and learnings. I always give you time at the end of a journey to write your insights down.

Treatment reaction

As shamanic journeys are very healing, you can afterwards have what is called a treatment reaction, which is when your body is releasing the old toxins and heavy energies that you started to heal and transform during the shamanic journey.

When this happens, you can feel tired, achy, emotional, and sometimes even experience viral-like symptoms. This is completely normal, and part of the healing process. So, if this happens, rest and trust that your body knows how to heal you.

Only move on to the next shamanic journey once this treatment reaction has settled, which can sometimes take a few days, and when you feel filled with energy again.

With all of this being said, let us take our first shamanic journey, into the four chambers of your heart.

Shamanic Journey
into Your Heart

· · · · · ·

Your heart is one of the first organs that was formed when you were a tiny foetus, as your developing body needed to be supplied nutrients through blood circulation. This means that your heart has been with you, from the very beginning, as a loving presence, nurturing you so that you could develop, expand, and blossom into whom you are meant to become. Your heart continues to do this throughout your life; with every heartbeat, you are lovingly guided on a mystical journey of healing, transformation, magic, and rebirth.

In this shamanic journey you will start to experience the sacred medicine found in each of the four chambers of your heart, but before we dive into the journey, let us do a quick recap of this medicine:

- **First chamber of the heart:** Here you will notice what areas in your life are "poor in spirit," so that you can take steps to release them and allow the *healing* journey into the darkness to begin.

- **Second chamber of the heart:** You now journey deeper into the sacred darkness, where you can start to *transform* what's meant to be healed.

- **Divine Source (lungs):** Here you journey up to the Divine Source—breathing in new inspiration, visions, and dreams from Spirit, thus breathing in the light of new life.

- **Third chamber of the heart:** As you continue to receive this magical light, you can allow this light to nourish your new visions and dreams. This *ignites your inner magic.*

- **Fourth chamber of the heart:** In the fourth chamber, you move through your own *rebirth*, so you can blossom—sharing your gifts, visions, and dreams with the world.

Below is a script of this shamanic heart journey, but I strongly recommend that you listen to it on **cissiwilliams.com/heart** so that you let my voice guide you through it; the recording is 26 minutes long.

The energy held in the spoken journey is really strong, so it will allow you to go much deeper than if you try to do the journey on your own. Listening to my voice helps you to drop deeper into your heart, while trying to do it on your own will most likely keep you stuck at the level of the mind, and you want to drop deeper, into your heart, so your heart becomes your shamanic teacher.

Make sure you can be completely undisturbed throughout the whole journey.

Shamanic Journey Into the Four Chambers of Your Mystical Heart

Sit in a comfortable position.

Close your eyes.

Sink into your inner stillness, into the light that shines in your heart, a light that is the eye of the heart, allowing you to see what Spirit would have you see.

Sink into this light now, deeper and deeper, and feel how this light becomes a portal into the World of Spirit.

Journeying into the World of Spirit

Take a deep breath in and, as you breathe out, feel how you journey through this portal now.

As you reach the World of Spirit, you notice you are in an ancient forest. The birds are singing, the sun is streaming through the treetops, the leaves are rustling in the wind, and the air is crisp and fresh, filled with the fragrance of wildflowers, pine trees, and soft moss covering the ground.

There is a path leading through this forest and, as you follow this path, deeper and deeper into the forest, you come to a temple that seems to be glowing from within.

This temple is a representation of your heart. It has four chambers and each chamber holds a different medicine. On this journey, you will explore what this medicine is for you.

Entering the first chamber of your heart

You now step through the entrance into this temple, arriving in the first chamber of your mystical heart. There is a golden divine fire burning in here, and the power of this holy fire starts to heal everything that you place in it.

This chamber helps you to let go of all that which is "poor in spirit," and it is the letting go that initiates your healing.

Notice now all that you are meant to let go of; all those thought patterns and behaviours that are stuck in fear, that are drained of life, that are "poor in spirit." Just notice what those thought patterns and behaviours are, so you become aware of them all.

Then start to place it all in this golden divine fire, trusting that everything you place in this holy fire is cleansed and healed.

Feel how you let it all go—as if you are shedding an old skin, an old way of being, an old structure you are now done with. Let it all go by placing it all in this healing fire.

Entering the second chamber of your heart

You now journey into the second chamber of your heart, where another divine fire is burning. Its bright hot flames glow with fierce compassion, and the power of this holy fire is that it transforms everything that you place in it into light.

You are here being met by the Dark Mothers, who are lunar goddesses, connected to the medicine found in the night, a medicine of fierce compassion that helps you transform old wounds into wisdom.

Notice now all the old wounds you sense are meant to transform and heal and, as you become aware of them, place them in the glowing flames of the fire.

The Dark Mothers start to remove old, stagnant energy from your energy field, placing it all in this divine fire. It is as if they are "combing" your energy field for anything that is heavy, freeing you from the past by releasing it all into the fire, where it is transformed into light.

Journeying to the Divine Source

You now continue your journey out of this temple, and you start to journey up, up, up, into the beautiful darkness of the night—up to the moon and the stars—up to the Divine Source, where you breathe in new light, new inspiration, new visions, and dreams.

Let yourself breathe in this new light, this expansion, this divine inspiration. Let it fill you up. Just breathe it in.

Feel how this light flows into your whole being—for every breath, let yourself be filled with light, with life, with gifts from Spirit. Let yourself receive all this new inspiration, for every breath you take.

Now you start journeying back down again, filled with all this new light, new life, new inspiration.

Entering the third chamber of your heart

As you journey to the third chamber in the temple of your heart, there is a golden divine fire burning in this chamber, a fire that looks like a radiant sun. The power of this fire is magic.

You are here being met by the Light Mothers, who are solar goddesses, all connected to the life-giving, nourishing light from the sun that ignites the magic of life.

Notice now how well you allow yourself to receive this new light from the Divine Source, bringing in new inspiration, visions, and medicine into you.

If you notice anything that stops you from receiving all of this, then hand that over to the golden divine fire that is burning here.

Just place all those old ways of being that prevent you from receiving into the fire.

The Light Mothers now start to remove from your energy field that which stops you from receiving the light. It is as if they are "combing" your energy field of anything heavy, freeing you from old fears that have stopped you from receiving the light.

They place all these old fears into the divine fire where they are transformed into light.

The Light Mothers now place their hands over your heart, sending the life-giving rays from the sun directly into your heart space. Feel how the warmth from the sun starts to melt the ice around your heart—open your heart to receive these warming rays now and let the heat from the sun in, melting away the ice.

As you let the rays from the sun in, feel the divine flame within your heart being ignited. This divine flame is like your own inner sun. Feel how it starts to burn more brightly, becoming bigger and bigger, melting what has been frozen—transforming it all into light.

The more you open your heart so your inner golden sun can shine, the more you awaken the magic of life within you.

Entering the fourth chamber of your heart

And now you continue your journey into the fourth chamber, where a huge orange and red bonfire is burning—a bonfire that holds the power of rebirth.

Notice all your thought patterns, fears and behaviours that stop you from sharing all the beautiful inspiration, light, and healing medicine you've received from the Divine Source.

Place all these thought patterns, fears, and behaviours into the bonfire, where they will be healed and cleansed and transformed into light. Watch as they all burn away in the glowing embers of the fire.

And now it's time for *you* to step inside this bonfire.

Feel how you step inside this divine fire of rebirth—and let it burn through you. Let it release you from all old fears, old thoughts, and old ways of being.

Let it burn, burn, burn through you—through your bones, your blood, your heart and your soul—releasing you from the hold of the past.

Let yourself just burn, burn, burn—and feel how, as you are burning in this divine fire, you start to move through your own rebirth, where you expand into a new version of you.

Be like the phoenix who rises from the ashes of the old, reborn in this divine fire, into a new expression of your soul's essence and beauty.

Now step out of the fire, reborn.

Notice what this new version of you looks like, feels like, and sounds like. A new you who is filled with new inspirations, visions, and dreams.

Now start to journey out of the temple and back onto the path leading through the forest, journeying back to the portal that leads into the light in your mystical heart.

Journey back through the portal

Take a deep breath in and, as you breathe out, feel how you journey through this portal, now.

Back into your body.

Back into the here and now, bringing with you the gifts, medicine, magic, and healing you've just received from the World of Spirit.

Take a deep breath in and, as you breathe out, open your eyes.

⌒

Take a moment now to write down your learnings.

Also write a letter to yourself, from your heart's wisdom. You can start the letter with the words:

What my heart wants me to know is...

Then just keep writing for as long as you feel intuitively guided to. By doing this you create space for your heart to start communicating with you. Then put the book down and give yourself time to digest the healing that has just taken place. Always give yourself at least a few days of rest in between each chapter as the shamanic journeys are very healing.

Mapping the Path

Grow deep roots to harvest rich fruit!
When your roots run deep, you cannot help
but bear the fruit of the Spirit.
— MICHAEL BECKWITH

The shamanic journeys in this book are based on two concepts: that our heart acts as our teacher and inner compass guiding us on our journeys; and that the Tree of Life provides the portal and map into the World of Spirit.

The Tree of Life also illustrates the importance of moving with the changes of the seasons, as the tree lets go when it sheds its leaves in the autumn, retreating into the darkness of winter, and then emerges reborn in the spring, and bears fruit in the summer.

The Tree of Life is a representation of our nervous system, which is illustrated beautifully in the World Tree from the Norse tradition, Yggdrasil.

Yggdrasil as a representation of your nervous system

In the Norse tradition, the Tree of Life is seen as the World Tree, Yggdrasil, which is a huge ash tree. It represents the human body, and especially our nervous system, with the roots connecting us with our ancestors, the branches connecting us with our thoughts and with spirit, and the trunk is our spinal cord, connecting us with our life here on earth.

An eagle at the top of Yggdrasil represents spirit, according to Norse scholar Maria Kvilhaug, in her book *The Seed of Yggdrasil*. A hawk between the eyes of the eagle represents the third eye so, anatomically speaking, this would be the pineal gland in the brain.

A serpent by the roots of the tree represents the kundalini energy. This is the goddess serpent energy, lying dormant in our root chakra, waiting to rise as we awaken spiritually.

In the awakening of the kundalini energy, we begin to remember this ancient feminine wisdom that lives inside of us. It is as if this wisdom lives inside the trunk of the tree, inside our core, in our nervous system. In the *Voluspá, The Divination of the Witch*, the Old Witch talks about the "witches within wood"—the wood being the World Tree. Here, she is talking about ancient powerful female beings within our core, meaning that there is an ancient "witch-within-wood" within your core. And she is the one calling us all to awaken.

Journeying with Freya into the Land of Ice

From my earlier work with shamanic journeying, I knew the importance of the Tree of Life as a portal into the lower world, upper world, and middle world, but I had no idea that it would also be a portal into all that was frozen within my psyche, helping me to heal deep wounds held in my ancestral lineage. That was only revealed to me a few weeks after my mum's funeral.

Mum's passing hit me hard, and I was filled with grief. But I also seemed to have many other toxic emotions surfacing, as if an old poison was slowly consuming me. My thoughts were filled with venom, and I would lash out at my loved ones. I knew in my heart it wasn't just because I was grieving. Even my husband gently pointed out that I wasn't being myself.

One morning I got up early and sat in silence on the floor in my living room, as the birds were gently singing to greet a new day. I felt so consumed by these toxic emotions that I didn't know what to do, so I prayed.

I closed my eyes and sank deeper into the stillness within my heart. As I was tuning into the stillness, the Norse goddess Freya appeared in my inner vision. She took my hand and journeyed with me to the Norse World Tree, Yggdrasil.

She took me along one of the roots of Yggdrasil, down into the lower world, to the Land of Ice—you will visit this place later in a shamanic journey in chapter five. She showed me that here in the icy landscape resided all that was frozen in my psyche—all the thought patterns, behaviours, old wounds, and ancestral patterns buried deep within my unconscious mind.

Freya explained that I was suffering so intensely since the death of my mother, because I had old ancestral wounding buried deep in my roots. This was causing me this intense discomfort, and I was meant to heal and transform it.

As I looked around this Land of Ice, I spotted a huge yellow snake. It was so big that it seemed to be stretching all the way back in time. I sensed that this snake was linked with an ancestral wounding and that the yellow colour of the snake represented the venom of the feminine— the backstabbing, wagging of tongues, and passive-aggressive attacks underneath the surface.

I tracked shamanically, with the eye of my heart, how this poison had been passed down the generations, from mother to daughter, going back hundreds of years. I could sense how my mother had been unable to heal this within herself, but somehow, she had buffered me from the full force of this venom while she was alive. With her now gone, this venom had started to enter my nervous system, changing me into someone I barely recognized. I realized that I was able to witness this huge yellow snake in my inner frozen landscape because I was meant to heal this, so I could stop the venom from being passed on to my daughters.

Freya took my hand again, and this time we journeyed along another root of the World Tree, to the Land of Fire. Here I met a goddess that was half-dark, like the midwinter night sky, and half-light, like the Swedish midsummer night's sun. She was the Norse dark goddess Hel. She told me that her light and dark represented the light and the dark of life, the day and the night, the summer and the winter, the full moon and the dark moon, and that she was a portal of death, transformation, and rebirth. A portal into an expansion of consciousness.

Hel journeyed with me, bringing her divine fire with her, to the Land of Ice. Through the glowing heat of the fire, she started to melt all that which was frozen in my inner landscape, or psyche. As it started to melt, the snake came to life, and Hel then brought it through her portal of transformation, into the light, so it too could be healed.

Hel and I repeated this process with all the other thought patterns and old wounds that were frozen in my inner landscape. We melted the ice through the healing power of her divine fire, until the Land of Ice had transformed into a lush, green oasis filled with light, life, health, and vibrancy.

Hel then came and stood behind me, holding a sharp object in her hand. Leaning gently over me—she is a giantess, so she was towering over me—she made a little incision over my third eye. She then continued to make a cut from my third eye, up along my skull, down my neck and all the way down my spine to my tailbone, energetically opening up my brain and nervous system. She then whispered to me: "Let it all go. Let all the poison leave your brain and nervous system so it can flow into my divine fire, where it can be healed and transformed."

As she said that, I started to relax, and all the old poison started to pour out of my brain and nervous system—like a dark toxic liquid—and into her fire. More and more poured out of me, and not just a liquid, but also crystallized formations that were all those frozen thought patterns and old woundings. For me, these crystallized formations looked like pus pouring out of my inner psychic wounds, worms from what had been rotting inside me, venomous snakes representing poisonous thought strands, and pieces of arrows and daggers from having been wounded by attack thoughts.

I just kept relaxing, letting it all ooze out of my brain and spinal cord, while Hel gently coaxed it out of my nervous system, placing it all into her holy fire. I felt myself getting lighter and lighter. I realized that what was now leaving was the old ancestral programming I had been carrying within me. It had been activated when Mum died, as I was now the oldest to hold it all. I felt such deep gratitude that I was being shown how to release this. I could allow it to be healed and transformed, and so avoid passing it on to my daughters.

Once everything had been released from my nervous system, Hel poured a liquidized healing light all over me, cleansing me fully.

Freya then took my hand and journeyed back with me to Yggdrasil. She explained that I could meet Hel at any time, to help me heal.

I did this exercise that Hel showed me—of opening my nervous system and letting the toxins pour out of me—several times per week for the next few months, as the relief I felt afterwards was phenomenal. Each time I did this process, I could feel more of that old poison leave me. As it was leaving, I started to connect with a deep source of ancient feminine power and magic within me, the ancient witch within my core, the "witch-within-wood." It was as if my mum's death was now becoming a portal of rebirth for me, where I was awakening the ancient wisdom found in my own roots and ancestral lineage.

You will later experience a similar process to what I have just described in the shamanic journeys in this book, so you too can heal old wounds and ancestral programming held in your roots.

Tuning into Your Tree of Life

Since the Tree of Life is a metaphor for our nervous system, it can help us notice if we have unhealed wounds in our ancestral lineage, or if we are blocking ourselves from expanding into who we are becoming.

In my shamanic energy medicine sessions, I work with the metaphor of seeing the nervous system of my client as a Tree of Life. I also do this on myself, so I can quickly scan how my nervous system is doing in this moment in time, and in relation to a particular life area. Your nervous system will change from day to day, and from situation to situation.

In trees, their roots connect, forming an underground web of roots, linking them with each other—very much like our roots connect us with each other through the collective unconscious mind, our past and our ancestors—in the lower world.

The roots on the right connect you with your masculine ancestors and the masculine energy within you—the doing, thinking, and planning side of you.

The roots on the left connect you with your feminine ancestors and the feminine energy within you—the intuitive, creative, and magical side of you.

You may find that your roots are healthy, or you may find that they are stunted, wounded, infected, or filled with ice (frozen thought patterns and emotions).

The ground water represents that which is nourishing your roots, and you may find that the ground water is healthy, or it may be poisonous and toxic, representing old wounds that need healing.

The branches are symbolic of your thoughts and what you are becoming.

You may find your branches are strong and healthy, or you may find they are stunted, sparse, or with something blocking them—thus something may be stopping you from growing and expanding into who you are meant to become.

EXERCISE for Scanning Your Tree of Life

Let us do a Scanning of Your Tree of Life Exercise together now, so you can get a quick overview of how your nervous system is doing. I would recommend you listen to me guiding you through this exercise (visit **cissiwilliams.com/heart**).

Initial glance

Take a quick glance first, noticing what your tree looks like.
Is it straight or leaning to one side?
Is it balanced or is one side bigger than the other?

Roots

What are the roots like? Short or long? Healthy or imbalanced?
Notice what your left roots look like. Healthy and strong, or

overgrown, stunted, infected, or frozen?

Notice what your right roots look like. Healthy and strong, or overgrown, stunted, infected, or frozen?

What's the ground water like that nourishes your roots? Notice the ground water on both the right and left side.

Branches

What are the branches like? Is there something blocking the branches from growing?

Is there something stopping the branches from receiving the light?

Notice if there is a difference between the right and the left side.

Wisdom from the tree

Ask the wisdom within your tree the following questions:

- What do I need to know and learn so my tree can be healthy and balanced?
- What do I need to change in my life? What do I need to let go of?
- How can I nourish myself, and my tree, more?

∽

Whatever you notice in your scanning exercise, rest assured that you'll soon be healing and cleansing your roots and your branches, with the shamanic journey at the end of this chapter.

Wisdom Teachings: Mary Magdalene, the Tree of Life, and the Seven Gates
• • • • • •

I want to share an ancient wisdom teaching that also mentions the Tree of Life. It is from one of the early Christian texts, called *The Gospel of the Beloved Companion*, translated into English by Jehanne de Quillan. In this gospel the beloved companion is Mary Magdalene, and at the end of this gospel, she goes to the apostles who are grieving after Yeshua's death. Yeshua is the name of Jesus in Aramaic, the language Jesus spoke. She tells them of the vision she had just experienced and what Yeshua had told her. She shares that he had shown her a vision of a great tree, with the roots going deep into the earth and the branches reaching into the heavens.

She describes how there are eight boughs upon this tree, each of them carrying different fruits, and these fruits can only be eaten if you are able to pass through each of the seven gates—representing the seven chakras—allowing you to ascend from one bough to the next. At each gate, you must free yourself from an aspect of the ego in order to pass through.

The bottom branches of the tree are so thick with leaves that no light can penetrate. Instead, you have to trust that the light is within you.

At the first gate, you must free yourself from judgment and wrath to step through the gate and eat the fruits of love and compassion.

At the second gate, you need to let go of ignorance and intolerance to step through the gate and eat the fruit of wisdom and understanding.

At the third gate, you have to free yourself from arrogance and deceitfulness (duplicity), to step through the gate and eat the fruits of honour and humility.

At the fourth gate you must conquer the illusions of fear to step through the gate and eat the fruits of strength and courage.

At the fifth gate, you need to reject the deceiver (illusions) to step through the gate and eat the fruits of clarity and truth.

At the sixth gate, you must come to understand who you truly are, and this understanding gives you access to the fruits of power and healing—the power to heal your own soul—which allows you to ascend to the seventh gate, where you find the fruit of light and goodness.

As Mary Magdalene received this vision, she saw her soul ascend, to be filled with the light and goodness of spirit.

Her soul became so filled with light that it turned into fire, and she flew upwards towards the heavens. Her soul dissolved into a radiant light, like the sun. In this light, she saw a beautiful woman, dressed in brilliant white. This woman extended her arms, and Mary Magdalene felt her soul being drawn into her embrace. In this vision, the Tree of Life is a pathway of healing the soul through the seven gateways (chakras).

At each gate, we are given a choice. Will we release the hold the ego has had on us, or will we continue to be trapped in its domain? As we release the hold of the ego for each gate—judgment, ignorance, arrogance, fear, and deceit—we receive the fruit there, the fruits of love, compassion, wisdom, understanding, courage, truth, and clarity. Embracing these fruits gives us access to the power to heal our soul.

This allows us to become filled with so much light that we become like a divine flame of fire, ascending up into the heavens, where we meet the full embrace of the Light Mother, who is radiant like the sun.

We are this Tree of Life, deeply connected with the earth, with our Dark Mother, through our roots. We also need to journey upwards, connecting with our Light Mother.

This wisdom teaching of Mary Magdalene and the Tree of Life reveals to us the pathway of ascension, up from the sacred darkness, through the seven gates, and into the magical light of the Upper World. In the wisdom teachings of Inanna (you meet her in chapter four) we make the journey of descent, through the seven gates, and into the sacred darkness of the Underworld.

We need to be able to both descend into the darkness and ascend into the light, because the deeper we can go into the darkness, the stronger our roots will be. The more we can ascend into the light, the higher our branches can reach, allowing us to receive even more of the light from the heavens—a light that nourishes the whole tree, including our roots.

We need both the darkness and the light; heaven, and earth, for us to grow.

In the shamanic journey at the end of this chapter you'll experience moving through these seven gateways, releasing the hold of the ego-mind, as you ascend the trunk of your Tree of Life (and in chapter four you'll experience the descent through these seven gateways into the sacred darkness to find the gold within).

The Chakra System

· · · · · ·

In the shamanic energy medicine I practice, we work with the chakras, which are energetic vortices, like energetic gateways, situated close to major important organs in the body. These energetic vortices change according to our thoughts, emotions, and inner energy. By working with them, you can start to release heavy energy, heal old wounds, and open up to receive the light of who you are becoming.

The seven main chakras are:

1. **The root chakra,** which is situated at the base of the spine and the pubic bone. It is the gateway to Mother Earth, and a portal that connects you with your roots, your ancestors, and your past.

2. **The womb chakra** (sacral chakra), which is situated four fingers below the belly button. It relates to your womb and ovaries, so it represents the very essence of creation. It is the seat of your magic, creativity, passion.

3. **The solar plexus,** which is situated in your upper abdomen (stomach area). It is linked with your digestion and adrenal glands (which sit on top of the kidneys). It affects how you express yourself, and how able you are in following your gut feeling (intuition).

4. **The heart chakra,** which resides in the middle of the chest (heart area). It is linked with your heart and lungs. It is the seat of your ability to give and receive love.

5. **The throat chakra,** which is situated between the head and the heart. It is related to your ability to communicate your soul's truth and express your dreams and visions.

6. **The third eye,** which is between your eyebrows, where your pineal gland is situated (the remnants of your third eye, which registers light and darkness). It helps you to tune into the invisible World of Spirit, and to see the light in the darkness.

7. **The crown chakra**, which is situated at the top of the head. It functions as a portal to the heavens and to who you are becoming, in the same way the root chakra functions as a portal to the earth and your connection with your past.

Let's dive deeper into each chakra and divide them into categories based on how they relate to the *lower world* (with the Dark Mothers), *the middle world* (dancing with the seasons of darkness and light here on earth), and *the upper world* (with the Light Mothers). At the end of the chapter, I'll take you through a shamanic journey in which you start to heal and cleanse your chakras and tune into your Tree of Life.

The lower chakras connect you with the lower world and with the Dark Mothers

The root chakra, which is located at the base of the spine and the pubic bone, is the gateway to Mother Earth and into the lower world. It is the portal that connects you with your roots, your past, with your ancestors and with the ancient Dark Mother, who is the bringer of life.

A healthy root chakra helps you to not only feel rooted in life, but also enables you to receive nourishment from life, so a healthy root chakra strengthens your immune system and inner wellbeing. It also helps you to manifest abundance, since all abundance comes from Mother Earth.

When you have an imbalance in this chakra you can feel disconnected from life, as if you must do it all on your own. You may start to distrust others, and sometimes even life itself, as if you have a deep fear that somehow you won't be able to have all your needs met. This can set up problems with chronic exhaustion, recurring infections, lack of money, lack of safety, and feeling that you don't belong.

When you tune into your root chakra (you'll do that soon in the guided meditation at the end of this chapter) and if you notice that it is imbalanced, you may find that there is a sluggish energy here, or that your root chakra is closed. You may observe that the roots going down to Mother Earth have dried up, or perhaps are weak, thin, overgrown, or even frozen. You may also find that the roots look different on the right (masculine energy connected with doing, structure, planning, and also your male ancestors), or on the left (feminine energy connected with nurturing, receiving, intuition, creativity, and also your female ancestors).

When you start to heal your root chakra, you reconnect with life, with Mother Earth, and with the wisdom and medicine from your ancestors. This helps you to feel safe, held, and nourished by life. Healing your root chakra opens the door to you feeling as if you are fully *living* your life.

One of the best affirmations to heal your root chakra is to say:

> *I trust that I am a daughter of the Divine Mother, and that I am always held, loved, and sustained by her fierce love for me.*

The womb chakra can be found four fingers below the belly button. It is the home to your magic, feminine creative power, passion, sexuality, and relationships.

It is linked with your ability to birth your dreams and visions, as the womb and ovaries represent the very essence of creation.

This chakra connects you with the Dark Mother, who is the powerful portal of death and rebirth, and whose cauldron creates new life. Your womb is your inner cauldron, like a holy chalice, that is in tune with the Dark Mother's ancient power of creation, magic, and healing medicine.

When you scan your womb chakra, and you notice it is imbalanced, you may find what feels like a block here, or that your womb is filled with an unhealthy, stagnant energy. Tune into the feeling here and ask what its message is. You may find old wounds, hard lumps, or "unborn" foetuses that represent unborn longings, dreams, and creative projects that never came to life.

When you start to heal your womb chakra, thus healing your inner cauldron, you connect with the wisdom of the womb, which is the wisdom of the primordial womb from and through which all life stems. This awakens your feminine magic, power, and fiery passion, so that you can birth your dreams, visions, and soul gifts into the world.

A great affirmation to heal your womb chakra is to say:

I am here to share my dreams, visions, soul gifts, and
magic with others. Let me be a conduit for divine love,
healing medicine, and feminine wisdom to flow through me
and out into the world.

The solar plexus chakra is situated in your upper abdomen (stomach area). It connects you with your inner spiritual warrior goddess, so that you can have the energy and willpower you need to walk your sacred path.

This chakra influences how you express yourself in the world. When healthy, this energy centre allows you to stay true to your own truth, and honour your commitments to yourself.

When it is out of balance, you can become stressed, as this chakra affects your adrenal system. An imbalance here can cause you to develop addictions, power struggles, and to lose your connection with your intuition or your gut feeling.

When you scan your solar plexus chakra, and you notice it is imbalanced, you may find stressed energy here—which can feel tight, tense, and on hyperalert. Or it can feel totally drained. Maybe something is lying over or around your solar plexus, restricting it? Or perhaps you can sense how your solar plexus is leaking energy, maybe because you give your power away?

When you heal this chakra, you connect with your inner spiritual warrior goddess, which gives you strength and power, so you can keep your commitments to yourself, have clearer boundaries, and know which battles to pick, and which ones to let go of. You become wiser in how you manage your time, energy, and focus.

This gives you more vitality, and allows your nervous system to be more at ease. You also connect with your divine inner compass, so that you can follow your soul's guidance—through your gut feeling—on where to go, what to do, what to say, and to whom. A great affirmation to heal your solar plexus chakra is to say:

I am always held in the Divine Mother's fierce love for me.
Through leaning into her love, I can relax, trusting that she
knows how to protect me, while guiding me on my path.

The heart chakra connects you with the middle world, and with the eternal cycle of darkness and light

While the lower chakras are of the earth, and the upper chakras are of the heavens, the heart chakra is the gateway between the two.

The heart chakra is situated in the chest (heart area). It is the portal that bridges heaven and earth, darkness, and light. This is your inner chalice that connects you with the middle world, with your life here on earth.

The heart chakra is the seat of your ability to love and be loved. When your heart chakra is balanced and healthy you can love deeply, forgive others and yourself, and feel safe to receive love. But when you have been hurt, you tend to close your heart.

An unhealed heart chakra can store emotions such as bitterness, loneliness, sadness, grief, and deep emotional pain, which can form an armour around your heart. Other crystallized formations can often be found here, in the form of daggers, thorns, swords, shields, but also glass splinters, hooks, stones, and a sense of frozenness.

When you tune into your heart chakra, and you notice it is imbalanced, just observe what it looks and feels like. Is it guarded? Closed off? Wounded? Caged in? Do you find any thorns, daggers, knives, and other sharp objects here? Any grief, sadness, and hurt? Just observe. Know that what you observe simply indicates past situations in which you've been wounded, and it is now safe for you to start to heal this. Your body will only reveal to you that which you are ready to heal and transform.

When you start to heal your heart chakra, you connect with your cosmic loving heart, a source of ancient wisdom that has the ability to heal anything. A beautiful affirmation to heal your heart chakra is to say:

I place my heart in the loving arms of the Divine Mother,
trusting Her love to be my guide today.

The upper chakras connect you with the upper world, and with the Mothers of Light.

The throat chakra is situated between the head and the heart. It is one of your psychic centres and is related to your ability to communicate your soul's truth, and to be an expression of the Divine Mother's wisdom in the world.

When there is an imbalance here, you tend to feel as if you can't voice who you truly are or speak your inner truth.

As you scan your throat chakra, if you notice an imbalance here, it may look as if the light here is diminished, or that something is lying around the neck and throat, restricting it, such as ropes or chains. Sometimes you may find that this rope or chain is attached to a heavy weight, as if you are trying to pull this weight forward, or as if it is dragging you down. As you scan this weight, you may discover that it consists of old wounds from the past, or "musts" and "shoulds," or expectations from others that are now holding you back.

You can also find stones and other objects in your throat chakra, or around the neck, representing chronic negative thought patterns that may be from this lifetime, from previous incarnations, or inherited from your ancestors.

When you start to heal this chakra, you begin to communicate your soul's truth clearly and authentically, making it easier for you to express your dreams, visions, and soul gifts with others.

One of the best affirmations to heal your throat chakra is to say:

I am here to be an expression of the Divine Mother that sent
me. As I let Her speak through me, I help to bring more love
and wisdom and healing medicine into my world.

The third eye chakra is situated between your eyebrows, in nearly the midpoint of the brain, between the left and the right hemisphere. This is the seat of your pineal gland, the remnants of your third eye, which is the inner eye that registers darkness and light.

Your third eye is your psychic antenna, helping you to see what your physical eyes can't see, thus enabling you to see the invisible World of Spirit, and to see the light in the darkness.

The third eye is the chalice that connects you with the upper world.

When your third eye is out of balance you become overly analytical, sceptical, judgmental, blaming, and linear in your thinking. As you scan an imbalanced third eye, you may find that the actual "inner eye" is closed or blocked. Sometimes the block is because of a crystallized formation in the shape of a stone, thorn or blindfold lying over the third eye. But it can also be experienced as a fog, dark cloud, or even as a poison, that obscures the inner sight. Other formations can be found here too, so always trust your intuition to what you see, feel and notice.

When you start to heal your third eye, you begin to trust your spiritual eyes more than your physical eyes. This heals your perceptual filters, so you can see with your spiritual eyes as you journey into the invisible World of Spirit. All the shamanic journeys in this book will help you practice opening up your spiritual eyes. A great affirmation to heal your third eye is to say:

I am willing to see through my spiritual eyes, so I can see the light that is always present.

The crown chakra is located at the top of your head and functions as a portal to the heavens, to the upper world, and what you are becoming, in the same way that the root chakra functions as a portal to the earth and your past.

When this chakra is out of balance, it can indicate a deep depression, disconnection from Spirit, a sense of isolation, or a fear of letting Spirit be in charge.

As you scan an imbalanced crown chakra, you may find that it is trapped by a lid, or something lying over it, such as a cloak, helmet, or that it's surrounded by a fog, like a brain fog.

When you start to heal the crown chakra, you begin to trust in Spirit, to trust that the divine always has your back. You know, deep within you, that you are an eternal being on this amazing journey through life. You are open to receiving inspiration from the Divine Source. One of the best affirmations to heal your crown chakra is to say:

> *Today I let go and let Spirit lead the way, trusting that*
> *Spirit knows the path that is for my highest good, and*
> *the highest good of all.*

How we work with the chakras in shamanic energy medicine

In shamanic energy medicine, we often work with the different levels of consciousness that exist in each chakra. Our chakras change constantly depending on our state of mind, and what is going on both within us and around us.

Your mind is incredibly powerful, and it has the ability to create wonderful experiences, which it does when it chooses love. Each time your mind chooses love, you feel happier and lighter, and your chakras will correspond accordingly.

But when your mind chooses to focus on fear, blame or bitterness, your mind starts to miscreate, leading to conflict, tension, and stress. This in turn affects your body, including your chakras. Over time, your body will start to mirror this negativity back to you, via various symptoms, aches, and pains. It does this to try to help you *awaken*, so that you can make a different choice.

In shamanic energy medicine, as you scan the energy field around the body, as well as the chakras, you may find crystallized formations there that have been created by chronic negative thought patterns. You can often see them with your inner eye, but you can also feel them with your hands, so you can feel dagger-like shapes in your energy field, chains around your ankles, a noose around your neck or a shield over your heart. These crystallized energies are a direct reflection of the thought energy that is active at that moment in your vibration. You can release these crystallized formations by removing them physically, using your hands and your breath—breathing out the heavy energy, while moving it away from your body, and giving it to the holy fire or to Mother Earth, where the heavy energy can be transformed into light.

Let us now do a shamanic journey, where you tune into your Tree of Life and your chakras.

Shamanic Journey to Cleanse Your Chakras and Tune Into the Tree of Life

• • • • • •

Introduction to the journey

In this shamanic journey you will tune into your Tree of Life, to strengthen your roots and branches, so you can be nourished by the sacred darkness and the magical light.

You will also ascend through the seven chakras (like the seven gates in Mary Magdalene's vision), releasing the hold of the ego-mind, so you can receive the fruits from each chakra. We will focus especially on releasing the various judgments and fears that may be blocking you from opening up to the feminine magic and power within you—as healing this will help you awaken the Wise Woman within.

This shamanic journey can be helpful to do regularly, to cleanse and balance your chakras and energy field.

I warmly recommend that you let me guide you through this shamanic journey. You can access the recording on **cissiwilliams.com/heart** (it is 37 minutes long).

Shamanic Journey to Cleanse Your Chakras and Tune Into the Tree of Life

Sit in a comfortable position, and sink into your inner stillness, into a light that shines in your mystical heart—a light that is a portal into the World of Spirit.

Journey through the portal into the World of Spirit

Take a deep breath in, and as you breathe out, feel how you journey through this portal now, into the World of Spirit, where you arrive in a beautiful forest.

Notice how you are like a Tree of Life, in this forest, with roots going down, connecting you with the earth, with the lower world, with the past and with your ancestors.

Your roots also connect you with the loving and compassionate Dark Mother, who is helping you heal deeply, so you can move through a transformation and rebirth.

Let your roots grow wider and deeper into the earth, into the sacred darkness, so they can be nourished and supported by the Dark Mother, allowing you to be anchored in life.

Now tune into your branches on this Tree of Life, and feel how they go up into the heavens, connecting you with the upper world, with the future, and with the Light Mother.

Let your branches grow wider and higher, so they can absorb all the light from the golden rays of the sun in the heavens, allowing you to expand and blossom into whom you are becoming.

Tuning into your roots and receiving the healing fire

Now tune into your roots again, and this time tune into the energizing life force from the Dark Mother—her fierce compassion, her lava—feel, see, and experience this as a river of glowing fire flowing through her core. Let this healing, life-giving glowing fire flow up through your roots and into the trunk of the tree, filling you with vitality, life force, and passion.

71

Root chakra

As this healing fire enters your root chakra, notice if there is anything in your root chakra that needs to be released, healed, and transformed.

Perhaps you find some crystallized formations here, or some heavy energy—whatever you find, let the fire transform it all. Just breathe it out, releasing it from within you and letting the fire burn it all, transforming it all into light.

Notice now all the judgments you have, of yourself and others, and perhaps also of the feminine magic and power within you—let this fire burn through them, transforming them into light.

As this has all been transformed into light, let the healing fire from the Dark Mother now bring to you the fruits of love and compassion. Feel how your root chakra becomes filled with love and fierce compassion from the Dark Mother.

Let your root chakra also fill up with life force, vitality, and healing medicine from the divine fire of the Dark Mother, strengthening and grounding you in her love.

Womb chakra

The divine fire now continues to flow up into your womb space. As this healing fire enters your womb chakra, notice if there is anything in this chakra that needs to be released, healed, and transformed. Perhaps you find some heavy energy in your womb chakra, or some crystallized formations. Whatever you find, let the fire transform it. Just breathe it out, releasing it from within you, letting the fire burn it all, transforming it all into light.

Notice where the ego mind is taking over, trying to use your sacred inner cauldron of feminine magic for its own needs. Let the divine fire burn it all, transforming it into light.

Notice your intolerance and ignorance of yourself and others, and perhaps also of the feminine magic and power within you—release it all into this divine fire. Let it all burn, transforming it all into light.

As this has all been transformed into light, let this healing fire from the Dark Mother now bring to you the fruits of wisdom and understanding. Feel how your womb chakra becomes filled with the wisdom and understanding of the Dark Mother.

Let this healing fire now fill your sacred womb space with creativity, passion, love, magic, and manifestation power.

Solar plexus

The fire now flows up into your solar plexus. As this healing fire enters your solar plexus, notice if there is anything here that needs to be released and healed, and transformed. Perhaps you find some crystallized formations or heavy energy here. Whatever you find, let the fire transform it all. Just breathe it out, releasing it from within you and letting the fire burn it all, transforming it into light.

Also notice your behaviour patterns when you give away your power, when you let others drain you of energy. Place all these behaviours into the divine fire, and let it all burn, transforming it into light.

Notice now your arrogance—where the ego has taken over—and also notice where the ego perhaps has taken over by being arrogant towards the feminine magic and power within you, and around you. Place all those thought patterns and behaviours into the divine fire, letting the fire transform them all into light.

As it has all been transformed into light, let this healing fire from the Dark Mother now bring to you the fruits of honour and humility. Feel how your solar plexus becomes filled with honour and commitment to your inner spiritual goddess warrior, and with a deep humility, where you are free from the ego's arrogance.

Instead, you are deeply connected to your soul's eternal truth— recognising that you are an eternal soul, a daughter of the Divine Mother.

Let this healing fire now fill your solar plexus with willpower and determination, with health and strength, so you can feel your spiritual goddess warrior's presence, helping you to commit to walking your highest path.

Heart chakra

The fire now flows up into your heart. As this healing fire enters your heart chakra, become aware of anything here that needs to be released, healed, and transformed.

Perhaps you find some heavy energy here, or some crystallized formations, maybe even a tightness, like ice around your heart. Whatever you find, just let the fire transform it all. Just breathe it out, releasing it from within you, letting the fire burn it all, transforming it into light.

Notice now how the ego traps you in the illusions of fear—witness all the thoughts and behaviours you do out of fear, instead of love. Place all those thought patterns and behaviours into the divine fire, letting the fire transform them all into light.

Now release all the illusions of fear the ego has trapped you in when it comes to your own feminine magic and power. Place all those thought patterns and behaviours into the divine fire, letting the fire transform them all into light.

As it has all been transformed into light, let this healing fire from the Dark Mother now bring to you the fruits of strength and courage, so your heart becomes fierce—like a divine flame burning so brightly, filled with strength and courage to choose love, to be love, to express love in the world.

Let your heart chakra become filled with the power of love, giving you the courage and strength that you need.

Throat chakra

The fire now flows up into your throat chakra. As this healing fire enters your throat chakra, become aware of anything here that needs to be released, healed, and transformed. Perhaps you find some heavy energy here, some crystallized formations, some tightness. Whatever you find, just let the fire transform it all. Just breathe it out, releasing it from within you, letting the fire burn it all, transforming it into light.

Let yourself notice all the ways in which you've been deceived—and place all those ways in which you've been deceived into the divine fire, transforming it all into light.

Also notice all the ways in which you deceive yourself and others, and place all those ways in the divine fire, transforming it all into light.

Now notice all the ways in which the ego has deceived you into not recognising the feminine magic and power that lives within you—and place all of those ways in the divine fire, transforming it all into light.

As it has all been transformed into light, let this healing fire now bring to you the fruits of truth and clarity, filling your throat chakra with the truth and clarity of who you are, so you can speak your soul's truth clearly, and give voice to the Divine Mother's wisdom in the world.

Third eye

The fire now flows up into your third eye. As this healing fire enters your third eye, become aware of anything here that needs to be released, healed, and transformed. Perhaps you find some heavy energy here, some crystallized formations, or maybe even brain fog. Whatever you find, just let the fire transform it all. Just breathe it out, releasing it from within you, letting the fire burn it all, transforming it into light.

Let the fire now heal your third eye, opening it, so you can see through the eyes of wisdom, so you can see through your spiritual eyes, seeing the truth of who you are, seeing with clarity the light of new possibilities, however dark the world seems.

Crown chakra

The fire now flows up into your crown chakra. As this healing fire enters your crown chakra, become aware of anything here that needs to be released, healed, and transformed. Perhaps you find some heavy energy here, some crystallized formations, or some tightness. Whatever you find, just let the fire transform it all.

Just breathe it out, releasing it from within you, letting the fire burn it all, transforming it into light.

Now open up to the heavens and let yourself receive the fruit of light and goodness from Spirit. Just open up to receive all this light and goodness—let it flow into you, into your crown chakra.

As you keep receiving all this beautiful light from Spirit, feel how your crown chakra starts to glow and sparkle, as if it is on fire.

Journeying up to the heavens

Through the flames of this glowing fire, feel yourself now rise, up, through the crown, ascending into the heavens, up, through the cosmos, up into the light of the sun.

Here in the sun, you meet the Light Mother. She is filled with a glorious radiant golden light, glowing like the sun. She embraces you and welcomes you home to her love, her eternal wisdom of who you truly are—that you are this light.

Let yourself be held in her loving arms. Let yourself receive her golden, nourishing, loving light for you.

The Light Mother now gives you a gift that will help you on your journey, so you can always be connected with her.

Notice what this gift is.

Notice what it represents and how you are meant to use it.

Journeying back to the Tree of Life

Thank the Light Mother for this gift, and feel how you now flow back down to your Tree of Life, bringing your gift with you.

Feel how you become the Tree of Life again, with your roots

going deep, into the sacred darkness of the earth, where they spread out, far and wide, rooting you in the earth.

Feel how your roots start to draw up nourishment from the sacred darkness—from the Dark Mother—and into you.

The Dark Mother now gives you a gift that will help you on your journey, so you can always be connected with her.

Notice what this gift is.

Notice what it represents and how you are meant to use it.

Thank the Dark Mother for this gift, and feel how you bring this gift all the way up, through your roots, and into you.

Let your roots continue to draw up the healing medicine you need from the Dark Mother—and your branches continue to receive the healing medicine you need from the Light Mother.

Feel how your roots ground you, so you can be steady in life—and how the light from the heavens fills you up with magic and the blossoming of new life.

You are the container of both the darkness and the light—you are the sacred cauldron through which the magic of life is expressed—*through* you, and extended out into the world.

Bring your hands into a prayer position in front of your heart.

And let us now say a prayer to the Divine Mothers of Darkness and Light, to the sun and the moon and the stars, to the earth and the heavens:

Dear Divine Mothers of Darkness and Light,
I surrender to you my path, my heart, and the essence of my being.
I'm willing to heal, and I'm ready to follow your lead.
So from this moment on, I will take a step back, and let you be in charge, trusting fully that you will guide me to the steps I need to take for me to heal and transform deeply, awakening your ancient wisdom that lives within my bones—the wisdom of the Wise Woman—so this wisdom can lead me forth into how I may best help to bring your healing medicine out into the world.

And so it is. And so it is. And so it is.
Blessed be. Blessed be. Blessed be.

Then thank the Divine Mothers of Darkness and Light.

Let us now prepare to journey back, into the portal in your mystical heart.

Journey back through the portal

Take a deep breath in and, as you breathe out, feel how you journey through this portal now, into the light that shines in your mystical heart.

Take another deep breath in and, as you breathe out feel how you come back into your body, and back into the here and now.

Take another deep breath in and, as you breathe out, you can open your eyes.

Take a moment to write down your learnings and insights you've received from doing this journey.

Also write a letter to yourself, from your heart and the Divine Mothers of Darkness and Light. You can start the letter with the words:

What my heart and the Divine Mothers want me to know
is …
and then just keep writing for as long as you feel
intuitively guided to.

By doing this you create space for your heart and the Divine Mothers to start communicating with you.

Then put the book down and give yourself time to digest the healing that has just taken place, before you move into the next chapter, where you will begin your journey of healing, transformation, magic, and rebirth into your mystical heart.

Part 2

Journey into the Sacred Medicine of the Four Chambers of Your Heart

The Chamber of Healing

When I let go of what I am, I become what I might be.
When I let go of what I have, I receive what I need.

— TAO TE CHING

Now that you've been introduced to your heart as your teacher and your Tree of Life map for journeying into the World of Spirit, you have prepared the ground to dive deep into each of the four heart chambers, for healing, transformation, magic, and rebirth.

As you embark on this healing journey, you'll uncover the inner mythic map you've previously used to navigate life, a map that had been formed by your old wounds, limiting beliefs, and ancestral programming.

This old map may have served you in the past, but as you start to uncover it now, you may notice how it's holding you back and that you are meant to let it go, which you'll do in the first chamber.

As you move through the four chambers of the heart, this inner map starts to change, so that by the end of this book, you'll have a new inner mythic map—a map filled with all of the positive resources, soul gifts, healing medicine, and feminine magic you have received through this sacred journey. This new mythic map will help you to navigate life from the Wise Woman within you, weaving your heart's loving wisdom into your world.

This is the beauty of shamanic energy medicine—we work with changing our inner mythical landscape, our inner map. And by changing this inner map, we change how we experience life, and come to see the world around us through a different lens.

When our inner map is negative, we tend to see the world through the ego's fearful eyes—and this often leads to more conflict, tension, and suffering, as the ego-mind will focus on how we are separate from others and life itself.

When our inner map is positive and filled with magic, empowerment, and healing resources, we tend to see the world through the "eye of the heart"—and this often leads to more peace, joy, and expansion, as the eye of the heart will focus on how we are connected with others, and with all of life.

Our journey through the heart chambers will help us to shift our perceptions, so that we can perceive through the loving eye of the heart, instead of through the eyes of fear.

Let us now begin our magical journey with the medicine found in the first chamber of the heart—*the medicine of letting go and healing your roots.*

Letting Go and Healing
Your Roots

• • • • • •

If we follow the flow of the blood, as it flows through the heart, then we begin our journey with the first chamber. This is the chamber where deoxygenated blood from the body is being returned to the heart.

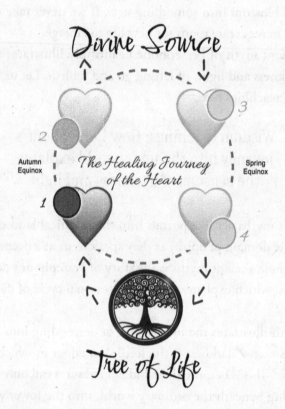

Figure 2: Entering the first Chamber of Letting Go and Healing

In this chamber (number 1 dot in Figure 2) we look at what is "poor in spirit."

What this means is that we look for all the outdated structures and identities we are meant to release, so we can create room for us to receive the light of new life later in our journey (when we journey to the Divine

Source to *breathe* in this new light of inspiration, visions, and dreams).

The first chamber represents the season of autumn when the trees start to shed their leaves, preparing to move through the portal of the autumn equinox into the sacred darkness of winter, so that they can be reborn when the light returns.

This means that the medicine of this chamber, which is the medicine of letting go and healing our roots, is vital for us to embrace in order to expand and blossom into something new. If we never take time to let go, then we never create room for new life to emerge.

The ancient myth of Persephone beautifully illustrates this sacred cycle of darkness and light, of letting go and rebirth. Let us investigate her wisdom teachings next.

Wisdom teachings: How Persephone's journey into the underworld explains the seasons of darkness and light

• • • • • •

Our ancient myths act like portals into the mythical landscape of our soul, into the domain of Spirit, as they speak to us at a deeper level.

One of these ancient myths is the story of Persephone's descent into the darkness, which explains the eternal seasonal cycle of darkness and light.

This myth illustrates the importance of descending into the underworld, as its sacred darkness is the fertile container in which we access our soul gifts. This is because these hidden treasures can only be reached by journeying beneath the ordinary world, into the lower world, into the domain of our soul.

A descent is usually followed by an ascent, where we bring up from the underworld newfound wisdom and soul gifts to share with the world. This is one of the meanings of the myth of Persephone.

The myth goes like this:

The ancient earth goddess Demeter loved her daughter Persephone so much that she could not bear to be parted from her. Persephone was very beautiful, and she attracted the attention from the ruler of the underworld, Hades. He wanted to make her his queen, but Persephone was never out of her mother's protective sight. Until one day, when Persephone was alone, picking flowers in a field. Hades saw his chance and abducted her into the underworld.

When Demeter could not find her daughter, she became so distraught that she forgot to tend to the crops, so they died. A famine broke out and winter befell the land.

Zeus intervened and tried to talk with Demeter, but she refused to let anything grow on the land until she recovered her daughter. Zeus persuaded Hades to let Persephone go under Hades' one condition that she would taste his pomegranate seeds before she left the underworld. Hades knew that if she ate something from the underworld, she would be forced to return to him, as anyone who had eaten something while in his kingdom could never fully leave.

A cycle of darkness and light, death, and rebirth

So, a compromise was made, and it was decided that Persephone would spend half of the year down in the underworld with Hades, and the other half with her mother. In this way, a cycle of darkness and light, death, and rebirth was set up. Every autumn equinox when Persephone descends into the underworld, her mother grieves, causing the leaves to fall and the darkness of winter to hold the land in a tight grip. When Persephone returns, reborn as the spring maiden at the spring equinox, her mother's joy causes nature to burst with life.

Persephone as inspiration for our own healing journey

In this myth, Persephone's mother represents the ripe corn of the harvest that nourishes the people in autumn, while Persephone represents the seed which drops back into the earth, where it lies dormant throughout the dark, cold winter. And then, when the light and warmth returns, the seed is activated and reappears as new life.

Persephone inspires our own healing journey, showing us how to let go of what has been and journey down into our own sacred depths found in the landscape of our soul, trusting that the seed of new life is already there, waiting for us. She also shows us how we can undergo a soul transformation and be reborn anew.

All the seeds of your future harvests already exist within you, in the same way all your future eggs existed in your body as a four-month-old foetus inside your mother's womb. Persephone had to let everything go for her to descend into the underworld, and likewise, you too are invited to release the old to prepare you for your journey into the second chamber of the heart, where you descend into the cauldron of transformation.

But before you can journey into the chamber of transformation, you have to embrace the medicine of the first chamber, which is to let go of the old, and begin your healing journey of transformation and rebirth, just as Persephone had to do.

Shamanic Inquiry Process to Let Go of What is Meant to Fall Away

We begin our journey into the medicine of the first chamber by looking at what is meant to fall away. Just as the tree sheds its leaves every autumn, you too must be willing to release the old for something new to be born. To help you identify what you are meant to shed, I will guide you through a three-step inquiry process.

STEP 1: See yourself as a tree in autumn

For this exercise, close your eyes, and see yourself as a tree, in the autumn. Notice the leaves that are meant to fall away. Each leaf represents an old part of your life—an old thought, behaviour, activity, or situation—that you intuitively know you are meant to let go of. Notice what it is that you are meant to let go of and write it down.

STEP 2: Releasing the old stories

Close your eyes again.

Notice now the old stories you have outgrown. Stories you've kept alive in the way you've given them focus, but now they feel old, stagnant, and lifeless, as holding on to them just keeps you stuck in the past.

Notice the old stories you are ready to release and write them down.

STEP 3: Journalling to help you release and let go

Continue to write down all that you long to release—frustrations, anger, bitterness, blame, guilt, doubt— all that you are ready to release and are willing to heal. At the end, burn all the papers you've written.

When I do this exercise, I feel how I energetically purge myself, from within, and out on paper, letting all I wish to release pour out of me. I keep writing and writing, until I feel I've emptied it all out. And then I burn the papers in a bonfire or with matches, holding the papers over the kitchen sink. And as I see the papers burn, I can feel the energy shift. The heaviness is transformed into lightness.

Never underestimate the power of journalling. It's a very effective way of releasing pent-up emotions and heavy energy. The key, however, is to burn the papers afterwards, or throw them in the bin, so you fully clear that heavy energy you've poured out onto paper.

Using two journalling books

Personally, I use two different journalling books, a practice you might adopt as well. One book is my *venting journal*, and I burn the papers once I've filled them. And the other book is my *wisdom journal*, where I write down all the learnings, insights, messages, and pieces of wisdom I've received during my shamanic journeys.

Now that we've discovered and released what's meant to fall away, let us tune into how you can heal your roots.

Heal Your Roots and Ancestral Lineage

The health of a tree is dependent upon the strength of its roots. It is the same with you, and your roots are linked with your ancestors.

Your roots hold your ancestors' wounding, and we all carry these wounds as many of our ancestors lived hard lives. This would have caused them to create limiting beliefs, such as being unworthy, unlovable, and unable to manifest their dreams.

Many were also persecuted, abused, killed violently, or suffered extreme poverty and despair.

When a wound remains unhealed, it becomes toxic and infected, creating something of a poisonous chalice that is passed down from one generation to the next. That is, until the day someone decides to heal this old wound. Through that healing process, the poison is transformed into a healing medicine, and this medicine can then be passed on to future generations.

Each ancestral wound you carry is a doorway into ancient wisdom within you. And as you step through this doorway, this ancient wisdom will guide you to the medicine needed to heal this old wound.

I experienced this myself when I was healing my coronary arteries.

The healing journey with my coronary arteries

After my heart attack, I was referred to a cardiologist (heart specialist). She thought the cause was my coronary arteries. I could feel the truth in this, as the coronary arteries' only function is to supply the heart with nourishment. If we see the body as a metaphor for the world, then the heart is a metaphor for us as individuals, meaning that a problem with the coronary arteries could indicate a problem with receiving nourishment for oneself. And I knew this was a personal theme for me.

After I had been to the cardiologist, I decided to journey into my coronary arteries, using my skillset as an osteopath and shamanic energy medicine practitioner, just as I had done with the four chambers of my heart.

I focused on four of the coronary arteries—two on the left, called the circumflex artery and the anterior descending artery—and two on the right, called the right coronary artery and the posterior descending artery. I decided to journey with the right coronary artery first.

I tracked shamanically (using my inner sensing and seeing with the eye of the heart, through which information is revealed to me, like an inner knowing) how the right coronary artery and posterior descending artery were linked with the masculine, like a river of blood connecting me with my male ancestors. This river was stretching all the way back in time.

My dad met me here, by this river. He asked me to notice the extent to which I was allowing myself to be supported by the masculine. As he asked me that, I realized that I had closed my heart from taking in support from the masculine. When I looked into this river of blood, I could see that the colour was quite dark, so not the healthy vibrant red colour I was expecting. I realized that the change in colour was due to old wounds and poison discolouring the river. Instead of nourishing me with medicine, this river was filled with a wounded energy.

My dad looked at me with such love and compassion. He knew that many of these old wounds and poison had come from how he had been towards me as I was growing up. He took me on a journey back in time, on this river of blood, showing me several events in my childhood when he had acted in a way that transferred the wound to me. At each painful event, I could reassure the younger me that all was well now, that I was here, that she was safe, and that we could let this old pain be released now.

I kept breathing out the energy of this old wounding, while in my inner vision, my dad and I kept clearing this river of blood of all the old poison, until it looked healthy, filled with a vibrant red colour—a colour that seemed to glow from within. In the journey at the end of this chapter, you will also travel back on this river of blood, so you can heal your ancestral wounds, and in this way receive the medicine for you.

I thanked my dad, and then I left this river and set off on my journey into my left anterior coronary artery, and circumflex artery.

I shamanically tracked how these coronary arteries on the left were linked with the feminine, like a river of blood connecting me with my female ancestors. This river was stretching all the way back in time.

My mum met me here, and she asked me to notice the extent to which I was receiving nourishment from the feminine. As she asked me that, I could feel how I had closed my heart to receiving love and support from the feminine, as if I didn't trust it to nourish me without wounding me. As I looked into this river, it was toxic, oozing with a dark poison, from all the back-stabbing women can do, underneath the surface—the wagging of tongues, the under-belly attacks. The river was green and yellow, with streaks of black in it. There was nothing healthy about it. No wonder I had closed my heart to receiving nourishment from *this*.

My mum said that the poison in this river was too deep, so she could not journey with me. Instead, the Dark Mother came. She took me back in time, on this river of blood, into my past, and into my ancestral lineage. We kept travelling on this river, and I witnessed how the circle of women had been broken as patriarchy took over, causing the women to be abused, suppressed and fearful of their own inner magic and power. As this happened, it was as if the women fell asleep to the truth of who they were, and instead of seeing each other as sacred sisters, they started to view each other as competition, as enemies. They turned on each other.

As we were travelling on this poisonous river of blood, I saw (with the eye of the heart) women being burnt at the stake, women being imprisoned, women being drowned. It was horrendous to witness.

I kept breathing out all this pain, despair, grief, and sorrow connected to my feelings as I was witnessing this.

The Dark Mother kept clearing the poisonous energy in the river too, with her holy fire, until the whole river was on fire.

I suddenly could feel a burning pain in my heart as we were journeying on this river of blood. I could sense how it was in the circumflex coronary artery. As I kept breathing out this pain, I was given images (from the eye in my heart) that showed how this artery represented the broken circle of sisters for me, and how the hard debris here represented unhealed wounds.

I kept on breathing out the pain, and the Dark Mother continued to burn and clear the river with her holy fire. As we did that, I could feel how I suddenly released a dark energy through my breath. I started to cough it up energetically, and in my inner vision this energy looked like a black poisonous jelly. I kept coughing this up, as we continued journeying further and further back in time on this river. I started to scream out all this pain and, as I screamed, I could feel this ancient rage flow up from deep within me. Rage over how women had been so abused, by patriarchy, and by each other. I screamed and screamed and screamed, and then I energetically vomited up a black slimy energy that the Dark Mother immediately threw into her holy fire, where it was transformed into light.

I heard a soft "pop" in my chest and then the pain in my heart suddenly stopped. I could breathe normally again, and I felt wave after wave of joy, lightness, and peace wash through me.

As I looked into the river, it was now a vibrant red, filled with light. I realized this river was now safe for me to be nourished by, as it was healthy.

I thanked the Dark Mother, and then I journeyed back.

∽

I did many more journeys into my coronary arteries, into this river of blood connecting me with my ancestors. For every journey, I could feel my heart getting healthier and stronger, as if my coronary arteries were being cleared out of an old, wounded energy from my past. And as they were being cleared and healed, I could open up and allow myself to be nourished by *them*.

One year after my initial visit to the cardiologist, I had my angiogram (scan of my coronary arteries), which revealed that they were all clear and healthy. And two years after that, I was discharged from the cardiologist unit as my blood levels were fine and various tests showed that my heart was now completely healthy. The only signs of a previous heart attack show up on the ECG, a test where they check the heart's rhythm and electrical activity. Given my tremendous recovery, they began to even doubt whether their original diagnosis had been correct.

I have no idea if the healing of my heart was due to all my shamanic journeys. It could all just be coincidence …

But what I do know is that by doing these shamanic journeys, I was able to heal deep wounds from my own past and ancestral lineage, and that absolutely had a positive impact on my wellbeing.

And most of all, this inner healing allowed me to *awaken* an ancient wisdom that was flowing in my blood—a wisdom from my ancestral lineage—the wisdom of the Wise Woman within.

I feel she is the one that called me to awaken, on that full moon in November, when she knocked very loudly on my heart, urging me to come with her, on this magical journey of healing, transformation, and rebirth.

So whatever challenge you are going through right now—be it physical, emotional, or spiritual—have faith that it is guiding you to awaken an even deeper wisdom within you; a wisdom that is your inner Wise Woman, and she speaks to you through the whispers of your heart.

Trust that your heart knows how to heal you.

At the end of this chapter, we will do a shamanic journey in which you can begin healing your ancestral lineage, healing the river of blood that connects you with your ancestors, so you too can receive their medicine for you.

Serpent Mother Medicine: Shedding the Old

••••••

As the first chamber of the heart is linked with letting go of the old, the animal archetype here is the Serpent Mother, the gentle healer that brings you the medicine of shedding the past, so that you can move into a new way of being, just like the serpent that sheds its skin to grow.

The Serpent was seen as a goddess in many ancient cultures, as she is closely linked with Mother Earth, and with healing our roots and our ancestral lineage, as she can travel into the lower world. Sometimes she appears winged, representing that she also can travel into the upper world.

The Kundalini energy—present within the base of our spine—is the feminine creative energy known as *shakti*. In the Norse tradition, this is represented by the serpent at the root of Yggdrasil, symbolising the feminine life force energy and, as she rises, she helps us to awaken our inner feminine wisdom.

In Aboriginal mythology, the Rainbow Serpent is a divine being that weaves through the world from Ayers Rock in Uluru, Australia, connecting various sacred sites, until it meets itself back in Uluru, thereby eating its tail. The serpent eating its own tail, the Ouroboros, is a sacred symbol that represents the eternal cycle of death and rebirth.

As the Rainbow Serpent travels, it is believed to form energetic veins that spread energy throughout the earth, much like acupuncture meridians in the body. In Britain these energetic veins are called *ley lines*, and in China they are called *dragon lines*. They look like serpents coiling around the world, similar to how our DNA, with its two helices, looks like two serpents dancing together.

Where these energetic lines cross, the energy is intensified. In some places, these energy culmination centres are so strong, many consider them to be the chakras of the earth.

The earth chakras are believed to be:

- Root chakra: Mount Shasta, North America

- Womb chakra: Lake Titicaca, South America

- Solar plexus chakra: Uluru, Australia

- Heart chakra: Glastonbury, Stonehenge, and Shaftesbury, England

- Throat chakra: Great Pyramid & Sphinx in Egypt, and Mount of Olives, Jerusalem, Israel

- Third eye chakra: Varies, but some believe it is currently in Glastonbury, Stonehenge, and Shaftesbury, England

- Crown chakra: Mount Kailash, Tibet

How patriarchy changed our view of the Serpent Goddess

The Serpent was revered in ancient wisdom traditions as a source of feminine wisdom, a great healer, and a messenger to the Great Mother Goddess. Then, as patriarchy took hold, this too changed. We see this change represented in the story of Adam and Eve in the Garden of Eden, where the Tree of Knowledge of Good and Evil exists, and they are forbidden from eating of its fruits.

In this story, the serpent whispers to Eve to eat of the fruit. Eve not only eats the fruit but persuades Adam to have a bite too. This causes them to be cast out of heaven and forever live in a world filled with death, suffering, and sin.

This story's impact on our unconscious programming is immense, as it has not only made us believe that serpents are evil and must be destroyed—a very common theme in stories focused on a man killing the serpent to "save" humanity—but it has also caused women to be seen as bad, evil, and untrustworthy. After all, it was Eve's fault we were all cast out of heaven!

What is the symbolism of the story of Eve and the Tree of Knowledge?

If we dive deeper into the different symbols found in this story, we can see how the Tree of Knowledge is a metaphor for the Mother Goddess, as well as a representation of our own body and nervous system, as in the Tree of Life.

The fruit is also interesting, as it is a representation of feminine wisdom and our soul's essence, as in the Norse goddess Idun's golden apples (you'll meet her in chapter 6) that contain the divine light-filled essence of our soul that gives eternal life. Even Norse gods have to eat Idun's apples to continue living.

The Serpent is a messenger from the Mother Goddess, so it is the voice of the ancient feminine calling Eve to wake up and EAT of the FRUIT of her own knowledge and wisdom, that is already present within her body, in her own core.

With this new interpretation of this ancient story, we can see that all that Eve is doing is hearing the call from the ancient divine feminine, guiding her to eat of the fruit of her own feminine wisdom and magic, so that she can awaken to the truth of who she is. And once she has awakened, she helps Adam awaken too.

How to relate to the Serpent Mother if you have a snake phobia

I am often asked how we can work with the Serpent Mother if we have a snake phobia. I totally understand this concern, as I have a snake phobia myself.

But although I have a fear of snakes, I have come to develop a beautiful connection with the Serpent Mother. She often reveals herself to me as a sweet-looking, light-filled winged dragon—there is a strong connection between dragons and serpents—as she knows I am more comfortable seeing her this way. And perhaps you may experience her as a dragon too, or as a light-filled serpent, perhaps even with wings?

Just stay open to how she presents herself to you, and trust that she is a great healer.

The Medicine of the Serpent Mother

One of the most potent medicines Serpent Mother brings is knowledge of when it is time to shed her skin, as the old one is becoming too tight due to new skin growing underneath. She then rubs her head against a hard surface to create an opening in the skin, so she can slide out of that old confinement. And she does that in one big, long "swoosh." She does not peel away one tiny piece at a time; instead, she decides it's time to let go of the *whole outdated structure*. And through her willingness to let the past go, she gracefully allows herself to be renewed.

In this way, the Serpent Mother shows us how we need to let go of the old, to give room for a new expression of longing to emerge through us.

The Serpent Mother brings a very soft, loving energy that assists you in releasing what no longer serves you. She also helps you to heal the body, just as she can free herself from scars and parasites when she sheds her skin.

INQUIRY: Serpent Medicine Questions

To tune into the medicine from the Serpent Mother, it can be helpful to write down the answers to the following two questions:

- Close your eyes and see the Serpent Mother, an ancient healer, and a goddess of light. You may see her as a beautiful Serpent, or perhaps like a gentle dragon. Let her reveal to you which old skins you are meant to shed—old skins as in old identities, old beliefs, old behaviours, old emotions, old limiting thought patterns, and old wounds and scars. Structures that feel like an old constriction, of which you long to wriggle free.

- Notice which old patterns seem to be the recurring themes in your ancestral lineage. These can be patterns of poverty, problems with relationships, addiction, the inability to break through old limitations, or any other way your ancestral wounds show up in your life or those of your loved ones.

- Notice what these old ancestral patterns are for you.

- Now that you have identified various old layers ready to be shed, the following shamanic journey will help you to actually shed these, and deeply heal your roots.

Shamanic Journey with Persephone to Release the Past and Heal Your Ancestral Lineage

• • • • • •

I will now guide you on a shamanic journey in which you start to release the past to heal your roots and ancestral lineage.

In this journey, you'll tune into your Tree of Life, noticing the leaves you are meant to release, and you will also meet the Serpent Mother, who will assist you in shedding the old, thus preparing you for your journey of healing, transformation, and rebirth.

You'll then travel into your roots so that you can start to heal your ancestral lineage, and you'll also heal the river of blood connecting you with your ancestors, so you can receive their medicine for you.

In this journey, the Dark Mother Persephone, the Queen of the Underworld, will be your journey guide.

I strongly recommend that you let me guide you through this shamanic journey. You can access it on **cissiwilliams.com/heart** (it is 37 minutes long).

Shamanic Journey with Persephone to Release the Past and Heal Your Ancestral Lineage

Close your eyes and sink into your inner stillness. Sink deeper and deeper, into the stillness in your mystical heart—where there is a light shining—a light that is the portal into the World of Spirit.

Journey through the portal into the World of Spirit

Take a deep breath in and, as you breathe out, feel how you journey through this portal now—into the World of Spirit, where you find yourself in a beautiful forest.

In this forest, feel how you become like a tree—the Tree of Life—with your roots going down into the earth, into the lower world, into the sacred darkness, and the branches going up, into the heavens, into the magical light.

The leaves on this tree are now in early autumn, representing that which you are meant to let go of.

Notice the leaves you are meant to release in your life—these can be situations, people, aspects of yourself, limiting thought patterns, and old programming. Just notice what you are meant to let go of.

And then let it all go—let the wind carry the leaves away.

Let the earth take the old, so she can devour it and use it as nourishment for something new to be born later. Trust that the new is always born out of the old, so just let her take it all.

Be willing to let it all go.

Deeper into the sacred darkness

Your tree now moves deeper into the darkness of autumn—and this darkness is creating a soft blanket that wraps around the world, like a loving embrace from the Queen of the Underworld, as she ushers you to retreat deeper into yourself.

Feel how you draw inward, deeper and deeper into the core of the tree—retreating from the outside world, going deeper into the stillness of the sacred darkness, into the loving arms of the Dark Mother.

Meeting Persephone

And now you see her, the beautiful Dark Mother Persephone. She is holding a flaming torch in her hand causing her dark eyes to glisten like stars in the night. Her long hair is filled with the wisdom of the sacred darkness, and her heart seems to be glowing, like a divine flame lit by fierce compassion. She has come to assist you on this journey of healing.

Persephone takes your hand, and together you start to journey into a tunnel that is taking you deeper into the lower world, deeper into the sacred darkness. After a while, you come to a holy fire. A fire that has the power to transform and heal and cleanse anything you place in it.

Releasing the old with the Serpent Mother

Next to the fire is the Serpent Mother, the ancient healer, who is shimmering from a radiant light. She is here to help you shed that which you are meant to let go of.

The Serpent Mother asks you to witness the old stories you've outgrown—as you witness them, feel how you breathe the energy of those stories out of your being, and into the holy fire, where they are being transformed into light.

She now asks you to notice the old skins you are meant to shed—old identities, limiting beliefs, outdated behaviours, stagnant emotions, and negative thought patterns. As you notice them, feel how you breathe the energy of that old skin out of your being, and into the holy fire.

This is a holy fire that has the power to heal, transform, and cleanse anything placed in it, so feel how you now step inside this healing fire.

Let the fire burn through you, burning away the old skin you have now outgrown. Let it all burn, so you can shed it all in one go, just like the Serpent Mother does. Feel how you let it all go, in one big "swoosh"—now.

And then you step out of the fire, feeling freer and lighter.

Healing your roots and ancestral lineage on the right

Persephone says it is now time for you to journey deeper into your past, into your roots, to heal your ancestral lineage.

She asks you to tune into the roots on the right, and together with Persephone, feel how you start to journey down into your roots on the right side of your body, going down along the roots that are connecting you with the masculine energy running through your DNA—so with the doing, the thinking, the logic, and the structure.

Travel back in time, along your roots on the right side, observing the masculine energy running through these roots. As you do this, notice now what it is you are meant to heal here today.

Notice the woundings, the programming, the beliefs, the ways of being that you are meant to transform and let go of here today, allowing you to heal your roots, allowing you to heal the masculine energy within you, so you can source for something new.

As you notice it, feel how you just hand it over to the Dark Mother Persephone, into her holy fire, which has the power to transform anything.

Release that which you are meant to heal through your breath, through you moving it out of your body, and out from your energy field, so you may want to shake it out, breathe it out, stomp it out, and perhaps even scream it out.

As you do this, feel how you release and transform all that old heavy energy along the roots on the right, healing the masculine energy within you—and let the Dark Mother Persephone help you.

Then feel, see, and notice how your roots on the right start to search for the healthy ground water, the ground water of the sacred divine masculine. Let your roots find this healthy ground water now.

As your roots find this healthy ground water, you meet a guide here for you, someone who represents the healthy divine masculine for you.

It may be an ancestor, a spirit guide, or a mythical being. Notice who it is for you.

Let this guide now lead you from this healthy ground water to a river, a river of blood that is connecting you with your male ancestors all the way back in time.

Your guide from the healthy divine masculine is here with you, as is Persephone, and you also have your divine fire with you, so you can shift and heal any heavy energy you need to transform into light.

Let this river now take you on a journey where you meet your male ancestors.

Let them show you what it is they want you to witness today, what you are meant to heal, what you are meant to transform in your ancestral lineage.

Just witness it, as you will soon start to heal it. But for now, just witness what is here for you to heal.

Now notice the toxins and poisons held in the blood of your male ancestors, all the fear, pain, and suffering. All the oppression and insanity, all the wounds held in the collective of the masculine.

Just witness it all and, as you witness it, feel how you start to bring in this divine fire—like a fire of light, healing, and cleansing—into this river, into these old fears and toxins and poisons, so it all starts to heal.

As you are witnessing this, you become the portal through which this can heal. Your male ancestors can be freed from this and be released into the light—whilst the river is being cleansed, healed, and transformed through this divine fire, through the help from your guide of the divine masculine, and the Dark Mother Persephone, and through you being willing to heal it.

Use your breath, use your hands, and use your body to release it all now.

Also use your intention, and the spiritual eye in your heart so you visualize all of this being cleansed and healed and transformed.

By doing this you heal and cleanse this river of blood from the old wounds, so instead it can be filled with healing, with medicine for you.

As your river is being healed—let this guide and your wise male ancestors—now give to you their gifts for you, their medicine for you, their strength and support and nourishment for you, from the healthy divine masculine.

Let them fill this river with all their gifts for you so this river can nourish and sustain you. Let the river be filled with so much light it starts to sparkle and glow from all this light, all this medicine.

Now notice how your roots on the right are reaching all the way down to this river of light, so your roots can be nourished by all this medicine from the healthy divine masculine, so your ancestral roots can support and nourish you.

Let your roots drink from all this medicine now.

And now come back with your awareness to your Tree of Life, to the middle of your tree.

Healing your roots and ancestral lineage on the left

Tune into your roots again, and this time tune into your roots on the left, which are connecting you with your female ancestors, with the feminine energy running through your DNA.

Together with Persephone, feel yourself travel down the roots on the left, back in time, whilst you are observing the feminine energy running through your roots, through your DNA—your creativity, your magic, your power to birth new life, and your ability to trust in the mystery of the divine.

As you continue to journey down the roots on the left notice what it is you are meant to heal here today. Notice the woundings, the programming, the beliefs, the ways of being that you are meant to heal, transform, and let go of here today, allowing you to heal your roots, and to heal the feminine energy within you, so you can source for something new.

Notice what it is you are meant to heal and, as you notice it, feel how you just hand it over to the Dark Mother Persephone, to her holy fire that has the power to transform anything.

Release it through your breath, through you moving it out of your body, of your energy field—you may want to shake it out, breathe it out, stomp it out, and perhaps even scream it out.

Feel how you release and transform all that old energy along the roots on the left side of you, healing the feminine energy within you—let Persephone help you.

Then feel, see, and notice how your roots on the left start to search for healthy ground water, the ground water of the sacred divine feminine. Let your roots find this healthy ground water now.

As your roots find this healthy ground water, you meet a guide here for you, someone who represents the healthy divine feminine for you.

It may be an ancestor, a spirit guide, or a mythical being. Notice who it is for you.

Let this guide now lead you from this healthy ground water to a river—a river of blood that is connecting you with your female ancestors, with the divine feminine, all the way back in time.

Your guide from the healthy divine feminine is with you, as is Persephone, so let them help you as you soon start to heal that which you are witnessing. You also have your divine fire with you, so you can shift and heal any heavy energy you need to transform into light.

Let this river now take you on a journey where you meet your female ancestors—let them show you what it is they want you to witness today, what you are meant to heal, and what you are meant to transform in your ancestral lineage.

Just witness it, as you will soon start to heal it. But for now, just witness what is here for you to heal.

Now also notice all the toxins and poisons held in the blood of your female ancestors—all the fear, pain, and suffering. All the venom and suppression, all the wounding and insanity.

Witness it all. As you witness it, feel how you start to bring in this divine fire—a fire of light, healing, and cleansing—into this river, into these old fears, toxins, and poisons, so it all starts to heal. As you are witnessing this, you become the portal through which this can heal. So, your female ancestors can be freed from this and be released into the light—whilst the river is being cleansed, healed, and transformed through this divine fire, through the help from your guide from the divine feminine and the Dark Mother Persephone, and through you being willing to heal it.

Use your breath, use your hands, and use your body to release the energy of all of this now. Use your intention and your spiritual eye in your heart, so you visualize all of this being cleansed, healed, and transformed now.

By doing this you heal and cleanse this river of blood from the old, so it instead can be filled with healing, with medicine for you.

As your river is being healed—let this guide and your wise female ancestors—now give to you their gifts for you, their medicine for you, their love and magic and feminine power for you.

Let them fill this river with all their gifts for you, so this river can nourish and sustain you.

Let the river be filled with so much light, it starts to sparkle and glow from all this medicine and light.

Notice now how your roots on the left are reaching all the way down to this river of light. Let your roots drink from all this medicine so they grow strong and become filled with life and vibrancy, helping you to trust the magic within you, where you dance in balance with the darkness and the light, birthing new life, new consciousness, into being.

Now come back with your awareness to your Tree of Life, to the middle of your tree.

Filling up with nourishment

Feel how your roots on the left and the right are supporting you, deep into the earth, connecting you with the sacred darkness, filling you with health, strength, wisdom, and medicine from your ancestors, and with a deep inner knowing that your ancestors are always here, helping you and supporting you.

Draw this nourishing medicine from the sacred darkness up through your roots—draw up vitality, healing, clarity, intuition, love, life force, magic, and all this healing, sacred medicine up through your roots, and into the trunk of the tree.

And as you are here now, by the tree, Persephone gives you a seed of light, the seed of something new that you are receiving here in the sacred darkness, from the Queen of the Underworld. Notice what this seed is.

Then place this seed within you, so you can hold it in a sacred space and nurture it until it is ready to emerge.

Now tune into the branches of the tree, and feel how they stretch up towards the heavens, opening up to receive the light from the sun, the moon, and the stars.

Let this magical light from the heavens fill you up, whilst you keep drawing up the nourishing medicine from your roots. Let the medicine from the sacred darkness and the magical light nurture your seed of light that you are now carrying within you.

Know that all is well and that you are on a sacred journey through life. Say goodbye to Persephone.

Journey back through the portal

Now prepare to journey back. Take a deep breath in and, as you breathe out, feel how you journey through the portal that leads into your mystical heart, bringing all your healing, wisdom, learnings, and medicine with you, coming back into your body, back into the here and now.

Take another deep breath in and, as you breathe out, you can open your eyes.

⌒

Take a moment now to write down your insights and learnings.

If you want to, write a letter to yourself, from your heart, and perhaps also from Persephone so they can share with you their messages for you.

You can start the letter with the words:

What my heart and Persephone want me to know is ...

Then put the book down and give yourself sacred time to reflect upon all the healing you have just experienced.

The Chamber of Transformation

The wound is the place where the Light enters you.
— RUMI

s we continue our journey with the flow of the blood, it now flows into the second chamber of the heart, which is bigger than the first chamber, and the medicine it holds is also more powerful—the transformational medicine of the Dark Mother.

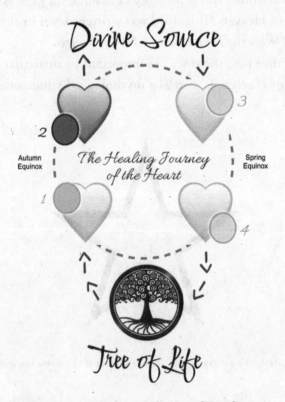

Figure 3: Entering the Second Chamber of Transformation

In this chamber (number 2 in Figure 3), we start to process all that which was "poor in spirit" by transforming it in the holy fire of the Dark Mother. This is where our shadows are transformed into light, and our wounds into wisdom.

The second chamber represents the season of early winter, where we descend into the darkness, into the cauldron of the Dark Mother, allowing us to undergo a deep transformation, so we can later give birth to new life once spring arrives.

Wisdom Teachings: The Descent of Inanna through the Seven Gates into the Underworld

● ● ● ● ● ●

An ancient myth illustrates the power of making this journey of descent into the underworld. This is the story of Inanna, the great goddess, and the Queen of Heaven. This story was written down in the Sumerian poem *The Descent of Inanna* over 4,000 years ago.

Before I dive into the story, it's important to share that Inanna, as the Queen of Heaven, is seen as a mythological representation of the planet Venus.

Figure 4: The pentagram, an ancient symbol of the divine feminine

Venus has an 8-year cycle, during which its movements form a 5-pointed star—the cosmic pentagram—an ancient symbol of the divine feminine.

It is also a symbol for paganism, with the top point representing spirit, and the other points representing air, fire, earth, and water.

Inanna's story illustrates how Venus moves across the sky, orbiting between the Earth and the Sun in a 19-month long cycle, where it changes from being the Morning Star, to then disappearing from view (as it is hiding behind the sun), and reappearing as the Evening Star.

This cycle follows the story of Inanna in this way:

- Venus as the Morning Star represents Inanna's descent into the underworld (263 days). During her descent she passes through 7 "gates" (monthly periods when Venus meets up with the Moon).

- Venus hiding behind the sun represents the time Inanna is in the underworld, where she dies to her old self (50 days).

- Finally, Venus being reborn as the Evening Star represents Inanna's ascent from the underworld (263 days). During her ascent she also passes through 7 "gates."

Now that we see how deeply rooted Inanna is in the feminine, both in myth and cosmology, let's dive deeper into her wisdom teachings.

The descent of Inanna into the underworld

Inanna's story begins with her hearing the call from the Great Below. She feels she is meant to journey down into the underworld to meet her older sister Ereshkigal.

She takes one of her faithful and trusted assistants with her, Ninshubur, asking her to stand guard, while Inanna journeys down to the underworld. She instructs Ninshubur to call for help if she has not returned after three days and three nights.

Inanna adorns herself with her crown, her jewellery, her bracelets, her shield, and her weapons—all of which show off her power and status.

She sets off alone, into the darkness of the underworld. When Inanna comes to the outer gates of the underworld, she knocks loudly. The gatekeeper, Neti, greets her, wondering why she is there. Inanna explains that she has come to visit her older sister.

Neti goes away to deliver this message to Ereshkigal, who is not pleased when she hears the news that her sister wants to enter the underworld.

She gives the instruction to Neti to bolt the seven gates of the underworld and says: "Let Inanna enter. As she enters, remove her royal garments. Let the holy priestess of Heaven enter bowed low."

In other words, Inanna can only enter the darkness of the underworld if she removes her outer adornments, which represent her outer ego-identifications. Thus, she is stripped bare.

As Inanna enters the first gate, her crown is removed. She asks: "What's this?"

Neti replies to her: "Quiet, Inanna, the ways of the underworld are perfect. They may not be questioned."

As Inanna descends deeper into the darkness, she comes to the second gate, where again she must sacrifice something. Inanna demands that the guard tell her what is going on. She wants to understand, but the guard replies that here in the underworld there are different rules. It is as if Inanna's mind cannot be allowed entry.

Inanna must sacrifice something at each of the seven gates, (representing the seven chakras) until she is stripped bare of all her power and identifications. At the very last gate, her royal robe is removed, so she enters through the last gate, naked, humbled, and bowed low, crawling to her dark sister, Ereshkigal, who is sitting on the throne.

The judges from the underworld are also here, and they pass judgment against her. Her older sister rises from her throne and gives Inanna the "eye of death," which strikes her dead. Inanna's body is hung on a hook on the wall, where she is left to rot.

When Inanna does not return after three days and three nights, Ninshubur senses something is wrong. She starts calling for help. She asks the Sky Gods for assistance, but they don't want to help, as going down into the underworld is against the law. She goes to the God of Wisdom, Father Enki, a god of the sea. He responds to her concerns with genuine care. He creates two little creatures—called mourners—from the dirt underneath his fingernails. He gives one of them the food of life, and gives the other the water of life. He instructs them to journey down into the underworld to meet Ereshkigal, and to respond to whatever she says with compassion and presence.

Because these two creatures are so small, they can pass through the gates without being noticed. They find Ereshkigal, who is howling in pain, grief, and suffering, as if she is in labour. They are compassionate and present with her. They don't try to fix her. Instead, whatever she says, they reflect back to her.

As Ereshkigal moans: "Oh! Oh! My inside!," they moan: "Oh! Oh! Your inside!"

As Ereshkigal sighs: "Ah! Ah! My heart!," they sigh: "Ah! Ah! Your heart!"

As they witness her pain with compassion, they moan and sigh with her, and she begins to heal. She thanks them and asks them what she can do for them. She is happy to give them anything, but all they want is to take Inanna's body back.

Ereshkigal agrees, so these two little creatures go to Inanna's body. They sprinkle the food of life and the water of life on her, which brings her back to life.

As Inanna ascends, she reclaims her adornments. So, when she reappears on the surface, she outwardly looks the same; but within, she is totally different. She now knows who she is without any of these old identities. She has faced death and been reborn. She has been deeply transformed by her experience in the sacred darkness. She has gained clarity and wisdom.

What is the symbolism of the story of Inanna?

In Inanna's story, she first hears the call from the Great Below to start her descent into the underworld, just as we hear the call from the Dark

Mother to make this journey of healing and transformation. She asks her trusted helper to keep guard above the surface, representing how we instruct our mind to keep an eye out for our safety, as we make this descent. But the mind cannot descend with us, as this is not a journey of the mind, but of the soul.

As Inanna descends, she is not allowed to understand the steps of the journey. Instead, she must surrender fully to it. This is symbolized in how at each gate or chakra she must give up one of her adornments, starting with her crown. Eventually she is stripped naked, and bowed low. For us, this represents how we must strip away the ego attachments, identities, and stories with humility if we want to encounter our soul at the depths of our own sacred darkness.

We cannot enter this sacred portal of death and rebirth without releasing the ego's hold on us. Just as the Serpent Mother must shed her skin to move through her renewal, we must shed our old ego-selves to be reborn.

Once Inanna has passed through the seven gates, she comes face to face with her shadow self—her dark sister Ereshkigal. As she approaches her sister, she is hoping to somehow be rewarded for her effort.

But her dark sister offers her none of that. She is filled with pain and grief and anger, representing those unhealed shadow parts of ourselves we don't want to see, so we push them down into the lower regions of our mind, into the underworld.

The underworld is the part of our psyche where we store everything we don't want to acknowledge—unhealed wounds, aspects of ourselves that are so traumatized we don't know how to deal with them, or parts of ourselves we dislike, so we push them underground, into the shadows, where they remain.

Ereshkigal is the dark sister aspect of us that knows all these parts that we have abandoned, rejected, exiled, and lost. They remain with her until we hear the call from the Great Below, when it is time for us to make this descent into the darkness, to meet our dark sister—our shadow selves—so that we can transform our shadows into light, our wounds into wisdom. Entering the underworld, Inanna meets Ereshkigal on her throne, where she is accompanied by the judges.

The judges we meet in our own underworld journey are emissaries of the Dark Mother, there to see through our ego illusions and lies. Ereshkigal strikes Inanna dead, representing how total and complete our ego death must be in our underworld journeys.

She is then hung on a meat hook, where she is left to rot, making sure there is no way for her ego to remain alive. She hangs there for three days and three nights, the same amount of time Jesus spent in the tomb before his body was resurrected.

When Ninshubur realizes something has gone wrong, she initially asks the Sky Gods for help. But they won't do anything, symbolising how the mind can't help us on this journey of death and rebirth. Instead, Enki, the god of wisdom and waters—representing the wisdom of our emotions—is able to help, through his compassion and ability to tune into the emotions. Indeed, it is our emotions, our profound compassion, and our grief—represented by the mourners—that are able to reclaim us from the dark and help our shadow parts to heal.

Enki's two helpers are like the two eyes of the Dark Mother, who can help us heal our deep wounds, grief, and shadow parts by holding us in compassion, by listening to our emotions, by witnessing our grief and pain.

We heal our shadows by meeting them with acceptance, not by trying to get rid of them. The more we push against them, the stronger they become, while when we meet them with love, they start to heal.

Ereshkigal's labour pains are a representation of how we undergo a deep birthing process as we enter the underworld, as it is the darkness that births the light. As the outer-world ego dies, our inner soul is birthing something new.

As Inanna is brought back to life, she is forever altered. She has now moved through a deep transformation and resurrection. This mystical process opens her up to receive the gold in the darkness—the gold being a greater expression of the truth of who she is.

As she ascends, she picks up all her old identities, but this time they don't define her. She can use them, but she is no longer trapped by them. She now possesses deeper wisdom, clarity, and understanding of her true worth. She has been initiated, taken through the portal of death and rebirth, thanks to meeting her dark sister.

As Inanna ascends, she is not only the Queen of Heaven, filled with light, but has also embraced the darkness of the lower world. This teaches us that to be whole we must marry the two, dancing with the fullness of life—embracing all the seasons of darkness and light.

At the end of this chapter, I will guide you on a very powerful shamanic journey where you too descend into the underworld, passing through the seven gates, releasing the ego-mind's prior hold on you. By doing this sacred journey, you begin to move through a deep transformation, transforming shadows into light, and wounds into wisdom.

But before we do that, let us look at how the Dark Mother helps us to heal our unconscious wounds.

How the Dark Mother Helps Us Heal Our Unconscious Wounds

• • • • • •

The Dark Mother is the primordial feminine darkness from which all life stems. Because she has been so vilified by patriarchy, many of us fear her, so we avoid journeying in to meet her. This effectively cuts us off from our deepest sources of fierce compassion and ancient wisdom.

I have come to understand that the Dark Mother is this healing, loving, divine presence, who is able to hold you in your deepest pain. She *knows*, she truly *knows*, how to assist you in your healing, as she understands your humanness, your emotions, and your wounds, and she also knows the loving truth of who you are. That you are a beautiful soul in a human body.

She understands how you so easily can become wounded by this physical reality you live in—as this world can be filled with so much suffering. She lives there, in the depth of your wounds, in the hidden areas of your psyche, holding you in a loving embrace to remind you that you are both human and divine. She gently whispers to you to let your love reach into these unconscious areas hidden in the shadows, so they can be transformed into light, compassion, and wisdom.

The difference between the sacred darkness and the unconscious darkness

It is vital to understand the difference between the sacred darkness and the unconscious darkness. The unconscious darkness is found in the deeper regions of our minds, hidden away from our conscious awareness. This is the place where our old wounds, frozen thought patterns, and ancestral wounded programming are stored. It consists of all that is unhealed within us, where love has not yet reached.

This unconscious darkness is not "evil"—just unhealed—but unhealed wounds can become infected. And this infection can spread, like a poison, into other areas of our lives. It can also be passed down the generations. This is how pain and dysfunctional programming can travel down the family line, until someone is willing to heal it.

The Dark Mother holds our unhealed wounds in a loving embrace

These unhealed wounds are frozen in time, and the Dark Mother is holding them in a loving embrace, creating sacred space around them, and waiting for you to make this journey of healing. As you make this journey, you are the one transforming the unconscious darkness into the sacred darkness, with the Dark Mother as your loving guide.

As you set off into the sacred darkness, trust that you will be met by the Dark Mother. She will gently guide you to witness the frozen wounds within you. The moment you witness these wounds, with compassion, they are no longer unconscious. The witnessing itself initiates the healing process.

She also knows you have the power within you to transform these old wounds into wisdom, and through that transformation, birth the light of a new consciousness within you. This is the light you can then share with others. This is how the poison passed through the generations is alchemized into a healing potion, becoming a source of medicine for your family line.

I will now introduce you to four different dark goddesses, all of whom are Dark Mothers: the Norse dark goddess, Hel; the Black Madonna; the Celtic dark goddess, Cerridwen; and the Greek dark goddess, Hecate.

Meet the Dark Mothers: Hel, the Black Madonna, Cerridwen, and Hecate

• • • • • •

All the dark goddesses are different facets of the Dark Mother. They come with slightly different medicines to help you on your journey, so you can call upon the particular Dark Mother you need most at any given time in your life. They all help you to heal and transform so that you can move through your own rebirth.

I will briefly describe four of them, and you'll experience their loving presence in the shamanic journey at the end of this chapter.

The Dark Mother as the Norse goddess Hel

The dark goddess Hel is from the Norse tradition. She is a portal of death and rebirth, helping us to let go of the past so that we can be reborn into something new.

Hel is a portal that guides you into a new life.

Her name, Hel, in Swedish means to heal (hela), whole (hel), sacred (helig), and something that is vaguely hidden (hölja).

Hel was worshipped as a powerful Dark Mother goddess for thousands of years. She was seen as a beautiful goddess, living in a place of rebirth, where her divine fire was burning. Through her healing power, she is able to move you through that portal from sickness into health, death into rebirth.

Half of her is dark, like the dark moon, and half of her is light, like the full moon. I see her as dark, like the winter-night sky, and magically light, like the midnight sun in the north of Sweden.

She is a powerful healer, releasing us from the poisons of our ancestral wounds and the toxins of the ego's thought system. She helped me heal deeply after the death of my mum by releasing poison trapped in my nervous system. She also helped me see what was frozen in my psyche by taking me to the Land of Ice, where she assisted me in transforming this frozen landscape through the healing power of her holy fire.

Tragically, patriarchy changed our collective perceptions of Hel, making her into someone scary and miserable—the ruler of Hell.

This is a typical patriarchal distortion of the powerful divine feminine, which tries to demonize it and compel us to push it underground. This has created an enormous wound and shadow in the feminine, where it has been suppressed, demonized, abused, and mistreated.

And of course, Hel wasn't the only goddess distorted by patriarchy. Mary Magdalene was pictured as a sinner and a prostitute, rather than the powerful mystic and representation of the divine feminine she actually is (you will meet Mary Magdalene in chapter eight).

The divine feminine is awakening now in many of us, because we are meant to heal these deep old wounds. We are meant to come out of the shadows and ignite the divine flame burning in our heart and soul, so we can go out and serve the world, sharing our heart's loving wisdom and healing medicine with others.

Hel will absolutely help us to release that which has kept us bound to an old perception of the feminine, so we can instead give birth to something new.

The Dark Mother as the compassionate Black Madonna

Another dark goddess is the Black Madonna. She is the Dark Mother who soothes your being in your darkest hours. She is the loving presence that rocks you to sleep and wipes away your tears. She is the gentle voice that whispers into your ear when you feel you can't go on any longer. She is the presence that has been with you in your deepest and darkest moments, in your despair and inner turmoil. She sees your light, even when you can't see it yourself.

The very first time I met the Black Madonna was in an underground chapel in Glastonbury, England—said to be the heart chakra of the world—and the experience blew my mind away. As I felt her presence, I recognized how she had always been there with me in my darkest moments, offering a loving embrace and accepting my humanness fully.

In that experience, the Black Madonna showed me what I needed to heal—it was as if I was sitting with her in a sacred inner sanctuary where a little fire was lit. She brought into my awareness people I needed to forgive, aspects of myself I needed to embrace, and actions for which I needed to atone. Wave after wave of pain, guilt, regret, and deep sorrow washed through me. For each wave, she was there, holding me, supporting me, accepting me, loving me, and giving me the sacred space I needed to heal my inner pain—similar to how the mourners witnessed and held Ereshkigal in her inner pain. Then the waves stopped, and I felt totally cleansed.

Following this experience, my research revealed more about who she really is. For some, she is the goddess of the underworld, dating back to pagan times. For others, she is the human side of Mary Magdalene, while others see her as an aspect of Mother Mary or associate her with the Egyptian goddess Isis. Whoever she is for you, she loves you, no matter what. Her loving guidance can show you how to transform your inner wounds into wisdom, by bringing them up into the light of your consciousness.

The Dark Mother as the Celtic goddess Cerridwen

The Celtic dark goddess Cerridwen is an alchemical goddess of healing, transformation, magic, and rebirth. She comes with her sacred cauldron, which is filled with Awen—the light-filled brew of inspiration, wisdom, transformation, healing medicine, love, truth, knowledge, and Spirit.

In this cauldron, she puts various herbs, plants, and healing ingredients, making a magical potion that will help you on your journey. What she puts in there will be unique to you, depending on what you need at that time in your life.

As you drink this powerful brew, you fill yourself up with her healing medicine for you.

The very first time I met Cerridwen, I was doing a shamanic journey to meet the Norse goddess Hel, who brought me to a dark forest, situated by a lake. Near this lake was a little cave, and inside it a little bonfire was burning. Over the fire was a cauldron and next to it was a beautiful woman, dressed in a dark cloak. It was Cerridwen.

She was placing various ingredients into her cauldron—moss, bark, pine needles, blueberries, lingonberries, cloudberries, light from the moon and the stars, sparks from the sun, and the velvety darkness of the night. She explained that the moss, bark, and pine needles were to strengthen my connection with my Arctic roots; the blueberries, lingonberries, and cloudberries were to help heal my blood; the light from the moon and stars were to connect me with the light in the darkness; while the sparks of the sun were to help me ignite my inner magic and feminine power. The velvety darkness of the night was the loving presence of the Dark Mother, to support me from within, so I could help to birth the light.

As I drank of her magical brew, I could feel how the medicine from each of the ingredients flowed into my body and consciousness. I felt lighter and more expanded, yet deeply rooted in life.

She then gave me a cauldron, filled with this powerful brew, and told me to go out into the world, sharing this medicine with others.

As I left the forest, carrying her cauldron with me, I witnessed how many came from far and wide to drink from this cauldron. And, as they drank, they were magically given a cauldron too, and invited to share its healing brew with others.

In the shamanic journey at the end of this chapter you will meet Cerridwen and discover the magical brew she is making just for you.

The Dark Mother as the dark goddess Hecate

Hecate is the Greek goddess of crossroads, the "in-between" spaces, and of beginnings and endings. She is also the goddess of magic and witchcraft.

You often find Hecate on the bridge to the spirit realm; holding two burning torches, so she can guide you onto a new path. She helps you make wiser choices so you can let go of the areas of your life that are ending, and embrace, with more power, the new path you are meant to walk—the path where you are expressing your soul's light, and sharing your gifts and healing medicine with others. Hecate can help you to see the consequences of both choices—holding on to the old or embracing the new.

She's often pictured holding a key, symbolising how she can unlock doors into hidden realms, as she is a liminal goddess who can cross between the underworld and our physical world with ease. She is also the one who accompanies Persephone when she returns to the underworld every autumn.

To me, she usually shows up holding a key that opens the door into the underworld, where she reveals to me something I need to heal. And at other times, the key opens a door onto a new path for me. In the shamanic journey we will do soon, you'll meet Hecate too, where she will give you a key that unlocks the door of new possibilities for you.

Let us now dive deeper into discovering our shadows, so that we can begin to transform them into light.

Discovering Your Shadows

The medicine of the second chamber of the heart helps us to heal that which we have suppressed down into the darker regions of our mind, into the underworld. This is where we meet our shadows, just as Inanna had to meet her dark sister, Ereshkigal.

When I started my healing journey, back in 1992, I focused initially on the light, so I focused on seeing the light in me and the light in others. This was the very first step on my spiritual journey, and I needed to stay here for quite some time.

But after a while, my soul called me to go deeper, as she knew there was more healing for me to do. And for that I had to journey down into the darkness, to heal the deep wounds held in the shadows of my psyche. This is when I started to hear the whispers from the Dark Mother, inviting me to journey into her sacred cauldron, into her holy dark womb space—to the Great Below, as in Inanna's story.

The Dark Mother has called you too. Trust that once you are in the underworld, the Dark Mother assists you in transforming the unconscious darkness into a golden light-filled medicine, which are all the soul gifts you are meant to share with others. You can only find these soul gifts by journeying into the sacred darkness. It is as if all these soul gifts are kept safe for you, in the womb of the Dark Mother, until you are ready to make this sacred journey of descent so you can retrieve them.

If I hadn't made my descent into the underworld, I would never have discovered the medicine and soul gifts I'm sharing with others now.

An important thing to remember here is that when you hear this call from your soul to descend into the darkness, you are not journeying into the darkness alone. The Dark Mothers will be there with you, every step of the way, as you face your own shadows and deep wounding. They will assist in moving you through a deep transformation, where the old shackles of patriarchal programming start to loosen their hold on you.

And as these old shackles fall away, the Wise Woman within you starts to rise. She has always been here, in the darkness, deep within your bones, like an ancient wise priestess, just waiting for you to make this journey of awakening. And, as she rises, you start to embody her ancient truth and wisdom. But now you don't just know it conceptually from your mind, you know it in your *bones*.

It is as if you awaken from a long sleep, a nightmare really, where you had forgotten that this ancient feminine wisdom lives within you, and that she is good, loving, and the giver of life.

The feminine is NOT evil, bad, or wicked, as patriarchy would have us believe—from the stories of how it was Eve's fault we were cast out of heaven, to how women's intuitive and healing powers were dangerous and deemed as witchcraft, and therefore punishable by death. And as you start to awaken, you realize it was all an insane lie, a distorted illusion from a twisted ego-mind that wanted to suppress this ancient wisdom that flows through your veins. You now realize that you have this sacred dark goddess medicine embedded within your bones.

You are the light—a light that is eternal and shines like a beautiful sun—and you are the sacred darkness of the feminine, a darkness that is the portal of death and rebirth. You are both.

As you recognize this, you are embracing both the darkness and the light, just as Inanna embraced both the darkness in the underworld and the light of heaven.

When you awaken to this realisation—that you are both human and divine, darkness and light—you start to birth a new golden consciousness into being. It is this new consciousness we are here to bring through, so that we can create a new world. And the Dark Mothers are the midwives helping us to move through this birth.

The key to birthing this golden consciousness is to heal the deep wounds hidden in the shadows, so that they can be transformed into a light-filled medicine.

Unhealed wounds fester in the shadows

As I mentioned earlier, when we don't heal the wounds that we have suppressed into the shadows of our psyche, they start to fester, creating an infection. This then spreads, like a virus that can be passed on.

This virus will start to infect our relationships, our thoughts, and our actions, until huge areas of our lives have been affected by this viral infection. And if we don't heal this, it will be passed on to the next generation.

The ego-mind, or our false self, is like this virus infection, and it thrives on our unhealed wounds. This means that the more our inner wounds fester in the shadows, the stronger the ego-mind becomes.

Developing spiritual antibodies

When the body gets invaded by a virus, it mounts an immune response, developing antibodies against this infection.

It is the same when you meet your shadows and take steps to heal them. Through your inner healing, you develop an inner spiritual immune system, which helps to clear up this wounded ego-virus infection. It is like you develop spiritual antibodies that helps to strengthen you. And once you've got these spiritual antibodies, you can go out there and help others heal too, as you are now immune to this particular virus strain. And then, when others start to heal, they too develop their own spiritual immunity.

This helps to transform the unconscious darkness of our world, where this wounded ego-virus has been able to fester. And then, bit by bit, we start to develop a spiritual herd immunity, causing the virus from our insane false self, the ego-mind, to loosen its hold on us.

When you take this journey into the sacred darkness, you are becoming your own wise healer, who can create spiritual antibodies within you, from healing these deep wounds. This starts to transform the unconscious darkness into light. As this light starts to glow, it is as if you are birthing your inner sun, from the sacred darkness within you. It is this golden light that you birth in the darkness that becomes the medicine to heal your world. At the end of this chapter, I will guide you on a shamanic journey where you start to transform your shadows into this golden consciousness, but before I do that, let's look at some of the ways shadows can show up in your life.

■ INQUIRY to Help You Discover Your Shadows

Let us start to unearth some of your shadows. For this inquiry process, I want you to write down the answers to each of the following questions.

- What do you judge in others?
  - Here look at what you dislike in others that makes you frustrated and annoyed. How you feel others are "wrong" and you are "right."
- What do you judge in yourself?
  - How do you make yourself wrong? What do you dislike about yourself?

123

- What are the parts of you that you try to keep hidden
  from others?
  - These are the aspects of you that you are ashamed of or fear,
    or that you believe would make others recoil in horror. They
    can also be the parts of you that you hide away, as you fear
    what the repercussions from others would be if they witnessed
    this side of you.
- What are you addicted to?
  - Here look at what thought patterns, behaviours, emotions,
    people, and substances you are addicted to.
- How do you avoid stepping into your power?
  - Do you do it by focusing on all your fears and worries, as that
    can keep you occupied for ages?
  - Or do you keep yourself bound to a limited perception of
    yourself, so you never have to step into your power?

Just keep writing down all that comes to you when reflecting on these
questions. Trust that you will soon release it, with the shamanic journey
at the end of this chapter.

Wolf and Raven Medicine: Protectors in the Dark

As the second chamber of the heart is linked with the darkness of winter,
the animal guides here are Wolf and Raven, and one of them also happens
to be my own personal *fylgja*.

In the Norse tradition, which is part of my ancestral lineage, we
acknowledge the presence of a fylgja (means follower) which often takes
the form of an animal. You have your own personal fylgja, accompanying
you throughout your life, and you may also have an ancestral fylgja. My
personal fylgja is a Raven, on my father's side my ancestral fylgja is a
Wolf, and on my mother's side, it is a Mama Bear.

The Raven and Wolf bring very powerful medicine, and by tuning into these animal archetypes, you begin to embrace this medicine for yourself as well.

Just as the dark goddesses have been vilified and misunderstood, so have the animal archetypes associated with them, such as the raven/crow and the wolf/black dog.

Over time, these animals started to be feared, instead of revered.

The Celtic dark goddess Cerridwen is associated with both the raven and the wolf. Hecate was said to be able to turn into a wolf, and she was often surrounded by a pack of dogs or wolves. And of course, the Norse dark goddess Hel has her Hellhound.

Wolfs and dogs are related, and for simplicity's sake I will refer to them all as Wolf. Ravens and crows are also related, being cousins from the same family of birds, *Corvidae*, and I will refer to them all as Raven. Just know that in the shamanic journey we'll do at the end of this chapter, you may meet a dog rather than a wolf, and a crow rather than a raven, so just trust your intuition on what is right for you.

Ravens are highly intelligent, as are wolves. In nature, they have a symbiotic relationship, where the ravens have formed social attachments with wolves, sometimes known as "wolf-birds." The ravens can be seen playing with wolves, and the wolves seem to like the company of ravens.

The ravens act as the wolves' eyes in the forest, helping them find prey, as well as warning them of danger. The wolves help the ravens too, by opening the carcass, making it easier for the ravens to take smaller chunks.

Ravens are associated with the archetype of the shadow, and in some Native American cultures, the Raven is seen as the creator of light, so the creator of all that existed before the beginning—the primordial darkness from which everything is born.

Raven is known as the messenger of the gods and goddesses, able to travel into different realms of reality, so it can help us on our shamanic journeys into the sacred darkness, being both a messenger and a protector.

In Norse mythology Odin's two ravens, Hugin and Munin, are sent out into the world to bring back information to him. They are symbolic of his shamanic eyes that can journey into different domains of reality. Hugin means "thought" and Munin means "memory," so Hugin looks at what is coming, and Munin remembers what is. In this way, Hugin is the shamanic eye looking at the future, what shall be, and Munin is the shamanic eye looking at what is, and the past.

When Raven shows up on our journey into the World of Spirit, they can help us by flying ahead, gathering information, and delivering to us messages of wisdom. They also act as guardians and protectors.

Wolves are also associated with the archetype of the protector, as they look after the pack. They are very social animals, forming deep bonds with each other. They educate their young, look after the old, and care for the sick and injured.

Wolf represents wisdom, wildness, inner freedom, and an ability to track that which is unseen.

When Wolf shows up on our journey into the World of Spirit, they may come on their own, acting as our protector and journey companion, but often their pack will be nearby, creating a boundary of protection around us.

Let us now do another inquiry process, this time tuning into the medicine from Wolf and Raven. Write down your answer to the following questions.

INQUIRY: Wolf Medicine Questions

- Close your eyes and see Wolf in front of you. Let Wolf now show you what old patterns in your life seem to be stalking you, patterns you now want to release.
- Let Wolf reveal to you how you are frozen, numb, or disconnected from your emotions, your body, and others. Notice what has caused this.
- Still with Wolf present, now notice how you run away from your inner pain. Perhaps by making yourself busy, blaming others, shutting down, escaping into your head—or perhaps by ignoring the pain completely, by pretending it is not there?

- Let Wolf show you where you are trying to rely too much on your own power, instead of allowing support from others (the support of the pack). How can you change this, so that you let yourself be supported by others?
- How can you take better care of your body, and your pack (your boundaries, as well as your loved ones)?

INQUIRY: Raven Medicine Questions

- Close your eyes and see Raven in front of you. Let Raven now reveal to you what you are unwilling to see in others. Perhaps you are unwilling to see if someone is being abusive, unkind, selfish, uncaring? Just notice what you are unwilling to see in others.
- Let Raven also show you what you are unwilling to see in yourself. Perhaps you are unwilling to see where you are being wounded and hurt, pretending that you are fine? Or maybe you are unwilling to witness where you are being bitter, blaming, abusive or too focused on you, too focused on what you can get? Just notice what you are unwilling to witness in yourself.
- Fly up with Raven into the air and look down on your life. Notice what it is from your past that stops you from moving forward.
- Also notice what it is that you keep chasing in the future, that stops you from being fully present in your life, in the here and now.
- Let Raven share with you the wisdom you need that will help you heal this.

I will now guide you on a shamanic journey where you descend through the seven gates into the underworld, transforming your shadows into light, and wounds into wisdom, so that you can birth a new golden consciousness into being.

Shamanic Journey Through the Seven Gates into the Underworld, Meeting the Dark Mothers, Transforming the Darkness into Light

• • • • • •

In this journey I will soon take you on, remember that the Dark Mother knows how to heal you. Trust that whatever wounding you surrender to her will be transformed and healed. The key is to be able to identify the wounding, so you know what to surrender, by searching deep within you for the thought patterns, beliefs, trauma, shadows, and behaviours you have that are based in fear. I will guide you through the process of how to do this in the shamanic journey.

And then, the moment you discover something that is not in alignment with love, you hand it over to the Dark Mother—through your intention, through your breath, through your willingness to heal. And as you do that, it is as if you are being held in her loving arms, and she says:

"My beloved daughter, I've been waiting for you to come home to me so you can heal, so you can transform deeply, moving through your own rebirth. You are ready, my love. There is nothing for you to do except to let my love in. Let my love in, as my love will heal you. I am love itself and you know it in your bones, so just let me in. And as you let me in, a light will start to shine within you that was always yours. This is the light the world needs."

In this shamanic journey feel how you let her in. Trust that she is the source of your wisdom, and that when you make this journey of descent, that you are healing an ancient wound in our human collective consciousness—a wound which separates ourselves from her loving wisdom. A wound that is now being played out in the shadows of our unconscious mind, creating conflict, chaos and suffering in the world around us—as most of the problems we see in the outside world are stemming from this disconnection from our Divine Mother.

You've been called to help heal this ancient wound. Have faith that the Dark Mother is supporting you every step of the way. She knows how to guide you to transform the unconscious darkness into light, the wounds into wisdom, so you can birth your inner sun, your inner gold.

Let us do this journey now, passing through the seven gates into the underworld, releasing the hold the ego-mind has had on you. When you are in the underworld, you will meet your shadow self—your dark sister. The Dark Mothers will be there too, helping you to release that which no longer serves you.

By moving through this journey, you start to transform the unconscious darkness into light, birthing your inner sun.

You will also meet the protectors in the dark, Wolf and Raven, on this journey. This shamanic journey is longer than the previous ones we have done (60 minutes), as the second chamber is bigger than the first chamber, so the medicine in it stronger.

I strongly recommend that you listen to this very powerful shamanic journey when you feel awake and filled with energy. You can access the recording on **cissiwilliams.com/heart**.

Shamanic Journey Through the Seven Gates into the Underworld, Meeting the Dark Mothers, Transforming the Darkness into Light

Close your eyes and sink into your inner stillness.

Sink deeper and deeper, into the stillness in your mystical heart, where there is a light shining—a light that is the portal into the World of Spirit.

Journey through the portal into the World of Spirit

Take a deep breath in and, as you breathe out, feel how you journey through this portal, into the World of Spirit.

As you arrive, you find yourself in an ancient forest—a magical forest filled with the presence of Spirit. It's night-time, and the dark sky is filled with twinkling stars. The moon is round and full, brightening up the forest with her beautiful glow.

Notice how you are becoming a tree—the Tree of Life—with your roots going down into the sacred darkness of the earth, and the branches reaching high up into the magical light from the moon, and the stars shimmering so beautifully in the darkness of the night.

Your Tree of Life now changes, preparing to retreat into the stillness of the darkness. The forest transforms into a beautiful, silvery landscape of frozen trees, with snowflakes gently falling to the ground, creating a soft blanket that wraps around the forest, like a gentle nudge from the Dark Mother to journey deeper into yourself.

Meeting the Dark Mother

Feel how you draw inward, deeper, and deeper into the core of the tree—retreating from the outside world, going deeper into the stillness of the sacred darkness. Feel how you are welcomed into the loving arms of the Dark Mother—the primordial feminine force who's here to help and guide you on this journey.

She welcomes you and, as you look into her eyes, you can see ancient stars shining from deep within them.

She takes your hand and leads you into a tunnel that's taking you down into her sacred darkness.

The Dark Mother explains that you will soon pass through seven gates, and at each gate you will surrender various ways in which you've been trapped by the ego's thought system.

Together you descend into the underworld.

First gate

You arrive at the first gate. In front of this gate is a holy fire burning, a golden fire that has the power to transform and heal anything you place in it.

The Dark Mother invites you to remove from your head a crown the ego-mind has made for you—a crown filled with poisonous thoughts of bitterness and blame, of self-righteousness and self-importance. All those toxic thoughts that make you feel superior

and better than others. In this crown, you may also find toxic
thoughts that make you feel less than, inferior, and unworthy,
as these are from the ego-mind too.

Feel how you put this poisonous crown down on the ground.

Look at the poison in it. Notice the thoughts that have formed this
twisted, toxic crown.

Now pour the holy fire into this poisonous crown. Let it all burn,
burn, burn.

Feel how this poisonous energy also starts to pour out of
your crown chakra now that the crown has been removed. As it
pours out of you, the Dark Mother removes it and places it into
her holy fire.

Let it all burn, burn, burn.

Let the fire transform it all into light.

The Dark Mother now takes your hand and together you pass
through this first gate, into a tunnel that is taking you deeper into
the sacred darkness.

Second gate

Now you come to the second gate, and in front of this gate is
another holy fire burning.

Here you are invited to surrender the ego's eyes. Feel how you
remove two eyes from in front of the energetic field of your
physical eyes—as if you are removing the faulty, insane perceptual
filters through which the ego views the world.

Place these two ego-eyes in the fire.

Notice all the toxic judgments, righteousness, and rigid thinking
oozing out of one eye, as it's being burnt in the holy fire.

Notice all the poison, blame, and attacking energy oozing out
from the other eye, as it's being burnt in the holy fire.

Let it all burn, burn, burn.

Feel how this poisonous energy is also pouring out of your
physical eyes—and as it pours out of you, the Dark Mother removes

it all and places it into her holy fire. .

Let it all burn, burn, burn.

Let the fire transform it all into light.

The Dark Mother now takes your hand and together you step through the second gate, into a tunnel that takes you deeper into the sacred darkness.

Third gate

You come to a third gate, and in front of this gate, another holy fire is burning.

Here you are invited to release from your throat chakra all the ways in which the ego has hijacked your voice, so all the attacking words, blame, and bitterness. Feel how you take this out of your throat chakra, placing it on the ground.

Witness the poisonous energy that is here. And now burn it in the holy fire.

Let it all burn, burn, burn.

Remove from your throat the chain and lock that has been placed on your soul's voice—your true voice. Place this chain and lock on the ground.

Witness how it has stopped you from expressing your soul's truth. Burn it all in the holy fire.

Let it all burn, burn, burn.

Feel how this poisonous energy pours out of your throat chakra and, as it pours out of you, the Dark Mother removes it all and places it into her holy fire.

Let it all burn, burn, burn.

Let the fire transform it all into light.

The Dark Mother now takes your hand and together you step through the third gate, into a tunnel that takes you deeper into the sacred darkness.

Fourth gate

You come to a fourth gate, and in front of this gate, another holy fire is burning.

Here you are invited to remove from your heart all the ice, all the armour, all the shields, and all the ways in which you've blocked love out.

Place it all on the ground, and let it all burn in the holy fire.

Let the ice just melt. As it is melting, start to breathe out the pain that's been trapped in the ice.

Let all the old wounds and grief pour out of your heart and into the holy fire.

Remove the attacking energies coming your way—the knives, daggers, and stones—all the attacking energies that have wounded your loving heart.

Place them all in the fire. Let it all burn, burn, burn.

Feel how this poisonous energy pours out of your heart chakra. As it pours out of you, the Dark Mother removes all of it and places it into her holy fire.

Let it all burn, burn, burn.

Let the fire transform it all into light.

The Dark Mother now takes your hand and together you step through the fourth gate, into a tunnel that is taking you deeper into the sacred darkness.

Fifth gate

You come to the fifth gate, and in front of this gate, another holy fire is burning.

Here you are invited to remove from your solar plexus all the ways in which your willpower has been hijacked by the ego-mind—perhaps by causing you to go into doubt, worry, procrastination, or sluggishness, as this stops you from following your soul's guidance, your divine inner compass.

Or maybe you've been exerting your will upon others.

133

Feel how you just let all of this go. Place it all on the ground and let it burn in the holy fire.

Let it all burn, burn, burn.

Feel how this poisonous energy pours out of your solar plexus, and as it pours out of you, the Dark Mother removes it and places it all into her holy fire.

Let it all burn, burn, burn.

Let the fire transform it all into light.

The Dark Mother now takes your hand and together you step through the fifth gate, into a tunnel that is taking you deeper into the sacred darkness.

Sixth gate

Now you come to the sixth gate, and in front of this gate another holy fire is burning.

Here you are invited to release from your sacred womb space, your inner cauldron, all your creations that have been forced by your mind.

Feel how you place your inner cauldron on the ground, and witness what's not meant to be there. Witness your ego-mind in there, trying to hijack your womb's creative power, trying to use your feminine creative power for its own agenda.

Witness other people's expectations in there, and your old dreams and goals that never came to be.

All of this is blocking your seat of magic and creation. Place it all in the holy fire, and let it burn, burn, burn.

Feel how this heavy energy pours out of your womb chakra and, as it pours out of you, the Dark Mother removes it all and places it into her holy fire.

Let it all burn, burn, burn.

Let the fire transform it all into light.

The Dark Mother now takes your hand and together you step

through the sixth gate, into a tunnel that is taking you deeper into the sacred darkness.

Seventh gate

Now you come to the seventh gate, and in front of this gate is another holy fire burning.

Here you are invited to release from your root chakra all the ways in which you disconnect from life here on earth, all the ways in which you stop yourself from feeling what's underneath, and all the old identities you know you are meant to shed.

Place it all in the holy fire. Let it burn, burn, burn.

Feel how this heavy energy pours out of your very skin and, as it pours out of you, the Dark Mother removes it and places it into her holy fire.

Let this heavy energy continue to pour out of your skin, purging you from within of all those old fears and false identities you are meant to let go of. Let them all just purge through you, through your skin.

The Dark Mother gently starts to peel your old skin away, your old identity away, as if she's removing from you your old robes, your old ways of being—she places it all in the holy fire.

Let it all burn, burn, burn.

The Dark Mother now takes your hand, and together you start to step through the veil that is the final gateway into the Dark Mother's sacred chamber.

Meeting Hel, Cerridwen, Hecate, and the Black Madonna

Feel how you pierce through this veil now. As you pierce through it you enter a birth canal that takes you deeper and deeper into the sacred womb space of the Dark Mother, into her holy cave in the underworld, where there is a little fire burning.

You can hear, feel, and see several dark goddesses arrive in this cave—they form a circle around you.

You see the Norse dark goddess, Hel; half of her is dark, like the dark midwinter sky; and half of her is light, like the midnight's sun. She is a portal of death and rebirth, and a great healer.

The Celtic dark goddess Cerridwen is here with her cauldron of magic and transformation.

The dark goddess Hecate holds up her burning torches that light up the right path for you.

And you can also feel the loving and compassionate presence of the Black Madonna. They will be your witnesses here in the Underworld.

Healing with the Black Madonna

The Black Madonna now steps forth. She tells you to hand over to her your grief, your deep suffering, and your despair, as she knows how to heal you. She's the loving presence that is always here, in your darkest moments, whispering to you the truth of who you are—that you are a child of the Great Mother, forever loved, forever whole.

Share with her now your deepest grief, suffering, and despair and hand it over to her, hand it over to the holy fire of the Dark Mother.

Healing with Hel

The Norse goddess Hel now steps forth. She invites you to give to her those old poisons which you are carrying in your body, in your nervous system, in your energy—poisons that are not yours, but from your ancestors, from the deep wounding held in the human collective consciousness.

Feel how Hel comes and stands near you, opening up your nervous system, by placing a little sharp object over your third eye, creating an energetic opening there. She continues to make an opening, all the way up to the top of your head, and then down your skull, neck, and spinal cord, along your whole spine—she is opening up your nervous system energetically.

She whispers to you—*just let go my child, let me take it, let me release you from these old poisons*.

Feel how all the poison, all the old programming, all the old toxins, and all the old wounding start to pour out of you, and into the holy fire of the Dark Mother.

Feel how it gushes out of you, pouring out of you.

Hel is gently coaxing it out of your nervous system, into the holy fire, where it is being transformed into light.

Let it all go. Let it be released into the fire, trusting that the fire transforms it all into light.

The dark goddesses are still standing in a circle around you. They tell you that it is time for you now to meet your dark sister— your Shadow Self.

Meeting your dark sister

And then you see her, your dark sister. She comes and stands with you here in this sacred circle. Let her show you all the unhealed shadow parts that you have shunned, denied, ignored, and suppressed.

Let all these wounded parts of you that have been hidden in the shadows reveal themselves to you. Let them show you how they got wounded and the pain they carry.

Let them express to you their grief and suffering. And as they do, just witness them, with compassion, with love, with acceptance.

Notice how these wounded parts start to heal as they are being met with your compassion, love, and acceptance. As they heal, they start to transform and glow with a beautiful light.

As they start to glow, they start to merge with your dark sister who also transforms into a golden radiant light.

She is your dark sister and, as you love and accept her, she is transformed into a golden light.

As you and your dark sister embrace, her golden light extends into you, so you too start to glow like a radiant sun.

As you keep embracing each other, the more love and compassion you give to your dark sister, the stronger this inner golden sun becomes.

Birthing your inner sun

With the dark goddesses here as your midwives, you and your dark sister are birthing your own inner sun—a golden sun that can only be born through the marrying of the darkness and light. In this golden light are all the soul gifts and healing medicine that you are meant to share with the world. Notice what these soul gifts are.

Cerridwen's magical cauldron

The Celtic dark goddess Cerridwen now comes up to you. She is holding her cauldron of healing, transformation, magic, and rebirth, and she explains that she's making a powerful brew, just for you—a magical potion that will help you on your path.

Notice what the ingredients are that she places in this cauldron, and how they are meant to help you.

Cerridwen keeps stirring in her cauldron. You can hear the brew bubbling away, and as you look inside the cauldron you see a radiant light shining from within it. This is a magical potion filled with light, inspiration, healing, and with the essence of life itself. It smells divine, with a beautiful blend of ingredients from heaven and earth, darkness and light.

Cerridwen invites you to drink this healing potion. As you drink it, feel how its healing essence flows into you, into your bones, into your blood, into your whole being—feel how it fills you up with so much light and life force that you are being transformed and renewed from within.

Hecate's key of new possibilities

Hecate now steps forth, holding a key in her hand—a key that helps to unlock your highest choices. As you accept this key, notice the doors this key will unlock, doors into new possibilities, doors into whom you are meant to become, doors into what you are meant to say YES to.

Enriched with all your gifts, and with this golden sun radiating from within you—say goodbye to the dark goddesses.

Starting the ascent

The Dark Mother takes your hand and, together, you start your journey back up, through the gates.

Seventh gate

As you arrive at the seventh gate, you receive a gift that strengthens your connection with Mother Earth and your roots. This gift awakens the wisdom in you where you know, deep in your bones, that you have the power to heal and transform your ancestral lineage and your bloodline.

Accept this gift and let its medicine flow into your root chakra.

Sixth gate

Continue journeying upwards, until you reach the sixth gate.

Here you receive a new cauldron of magic and transformation. Notice the medicine that it brings for you, a medicine that strengthens your magic and feminine power, helping you to birth something new into being.

Accept this cauldron and let its medicine flow into your womb chakra.

Fifth gate

Continue journeying upwards, until you reach the fifth gate.

Here you receive a gift that strengthens your connection with your soul's compass, so you can have strong boundaries, strong willpower, and be committed to following your soul's path.

Accept this gift and let its medicine flow into your solar plexus.

Fourth gate

Continue journeying upwards, until you reach the fourth gate.

Here you receive a gift that strengthens your connection with your loving heart, a love that is so fierce that it burns like a divine flame, brightening up the world.

Accept this gift and let its medicine flow into your heart chakra.

Third gate

Continue journeying upwards, until you reach the third gate.

Here you receive a gift that strengthens your ability to express your soul's voice, so you can share your soul's truth, power, and magic, through your voice.

Accept this gift and let its medicine flow into your throat chakra.

Second gate

Continue journeying upwards, until you reach the second gate.

Here you receive a gift that strengthens your ability to see through the eyes of love and wisdom, activating your third eye, so you can see that which your soul wants you to see.

Accept this gift and let its medicine flow into your third eye.

First gate

Continue journeying upwards, until you reach the first gate.

Here you receive a gift that strengthens your connection with the light of the heavens, helping you hear, see, and feel and just know Spirit's guidance for you.

Accept this gift and let its medicine flow into your crown chakra.

The path in the forest, meeting Wolf and Raven

Enriched with all your gifts you now journey all the way back to the ancient forest.

The moon is still shining, and the stars are shimmering like diamonds in the dark sky.

You see a majestic wolf and a wise raven come toward you.
Let them share with you the medicine they bring to you, and how they support, protect, and guide you on your journey.

Embrace the medicine from Wolf and Raven and thank them for being here with you, as Animal Guides in the Spirit World.

Becoming the Tree of Life

Notice how you become like this Tree of Life again, with your roots going deep, deep into the earth, and your branches reaching high, high, up into the light from the heavens.

Even though the tree and the forest appear the same as at the beginning of your journey, you know you are deeply transformed. You are now enriched with all your gifts. Within you, a golden light is shining—a light that contains all the seeds of the soul gifts and healing medicine you are here to share with your world.

You feel the presence of the Dark Mother deep within your core, like a loving mother, supporting you from within.

And you know it's time for you to journey back.

Journey back through the portal

Take a deep breath in and, as you breathe out, feel how you journey through the portal now, coming back into your body, back into the here and now.

Take another deep breath in and, as you breathe out, you can open your eyes.

⌒

Take a moment now to write down your learnings and insights from this journey.

If you want to, write a letter to yourself, from your heart, and perhaps also from the Dark Mothers so they can share with you their messages for you.

You can start the letter with the words:

What my heart and the Dark Mothers want me to know is ...

Then put the book down and give yourself sacred time to reflect upon all the healing you have just experienced.

Returning to Source

Only from the heart can you touch the sky.
— RUMI

As we continue our journey, following the flow of the blood, it now flows up to the lungs, where the blood goes to become oxygenated.

The lungs look a bit like a Cosmic Angel, *breathing in Spirit*, filling you with the light of new inspiration, visions, dreams, gifts, blessings, and nourishment.

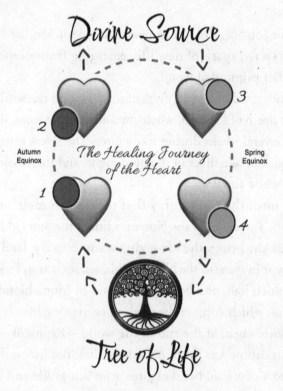

Figure 5: Entering the Lungs and Breathing in the light from the Divine Source

The lungs are a representation of the Divine Source, where the light-filled seeds of what's meant to be born already exist.

As you *breathe* this light in, you become pregnant with the seeds of new life, so you can later birth them through you. This is how you bring the light of the new from the Divine Source first into you, and then out into the world.

This corresponds to the seasons of the year—this time the Winter Solstice when the light is being reborn in the darkness. This returning light is the light-filled seeds of new life. And the flow of the blood reveals to us that what happens every year in nature, also happens within our bodies, with every heartbeat.

Wisdom Teachings: Birthing the Light from the Darkest Night

● ● ● ● ● ●

At the winter solstice, the sun is reborn. It is as if Mother Night gives birth to the sacred spark of new life, emerging from deep within the darkness of her primordial womb.

This is illustrated in several myths found around the world.

In the far north of Lapland, where my ancestors are from, the sun does not rise for several weeks during midwinter. The rivers turn to ice, the frosty trees glisten like silver in the moonlight, and the whole landscape is dusted in white snow.

It is not until the sun returns that the ice can melt, and life can flourish again. Therefore, in the Norse tradition, the Sun Goddess is very important, as she brings the life-giving warmth to the land. Her solar qualities appear in some of the Norse goddesses, such as in Freya's flaming necklace, golden hair, and golden tears, and in Idun's blonde hair and golden apples, which contain the seeds of everlasting life.

In the Norse sagas, at the end of the world—Ragnarök—the world is engulfed in darkness as the Sun Goddess dies. But before she dies, she gives birth to a new sun, her daughter, who brings life and light into a new world.

The birth of a divine child in the middle of the darkness is something that appears in other traditions as well.

The Egyptian goddess Isis mourned the death of her husband Osiris, whose dismembered body pieces were scattered in the underworld. Isis had great magical powers, so she managed to retrieve his body parts, bringing her husband back to life. They made love and Isis fell pregnant. Their son, Horus, a sun god, was born around the Winter Solstice—just as the light is being born on this day in the middle of the darkness.

Likewise, in Christianity, Jesus' birth to the Virgin Mary, is celebrated on December 25, so very close to the Winter Solstice. His birth symbolizes the light of the world being born in the middle of the darkness.

The concept of a Divine Virgin Mother who births a Divine Child is a metaphor for how we can become pregnant with the light-filled seeds of new dreams from the Divine Source and then—through our own feminine creative powers—birth these dreams into the world.

The midwinter solstice is the season for receiving these new dreams, and the lungs are the place where our blood becomes filled with all this new expansion of life.

Through us breathing it in, we are breathing in spirit (inspiration).

In many ancient wisdom traditions, such as the Norse and Celtic, this time of year is referred to as "dreamtime," as this is the time we start to receive the light of our new dreams from the Divine Source. And then we can work with the Spirit Weavers to help weave these dreams into being.

Weaving Your Dreams Into Being with the Spirit Weavers
• • • • • •

As we embrace the returning light, breathing in all these new dreams, visions, and inspiration, we have to learn how to weave this light into being. Many ancient traditions talk about weaving a new life into creation, such as the Hopi Indian myth about Spider Grandmother who, through weaving her web, thought the world itself into being. She is often seen as the Earth Goddess.

The Navajos talk about Spider Woman, seeing her as the first weaver, who could bring order and form, balance, and beauty, to what was originally chaos.

The idea of spinning and weaving is also found in other places in the world, such as the Ancient Egyptian Goddess, Neith, who was believed to have woven the whole world into existence, or the Hindu Goddess Maya, who is the spinner of magic, fate, and the illusory nature of appearances, helping us to understand that not all things are as they appear to be.

In the Celtic tradition, we find Arianrhod, the goddess of the moon and the stars, and the spirit weaver of cosmic time, magic, fate, and rebirth. She spins the silver wheel, which is the moon itself—so a wheel that governs all seasons, including the seasons of your life.

In Greek Mythology we have the three fates—Clotho, Lachesis, and Atropos. Clotho would spin the web of life, Lachesis would measure the thread of life for each person, and Atropos would choose the way in which each person died.

The three norns are archetypes of time

In Norse mythology we find the three norns. They are primordial beings, who are archetypes of time—past, present, and future. They live at the Well of Urd, also called the Well of Origin. In this well, you can see everything that has ever been, and the future that is unfolding.

Here at this well, the three norns weave the cosmic web, the web of life in which everything is embedded.

The World Tree Yggdrasil also grows from this well, and the norns use the healing water from the well to nourish the tree.

The norn of the past, Urd, is the oldest. Her name means "origin." She is very old, like a dark primordial being who births life itself. She is a Dark Mother who helps you heal your past, and therefore she is connected with the lower world and the sacred darkness.

The norn of the present, Verdandi, helps you to become aware of how you are showing up in the now, and therefore she is connected with the middle world, with your life here now, helping you to dance with the seasons of darkness and light. The norn of the future, Skuld, is a Light Mother, helping you to become aware of what you are bringing into your future, by showing you what is possible when you say YES to what lights you up.

The name Skuld means "debt" in Swedish. It also means "that which shall be." In this way, she is showing us that if we don't heal our past, we end up dragging our past with us into the present. We then show up from this wounded energy, spreading it into our thoughts, actions, and relationships. Plus, our unhealed wounds drain us of life energy, resulting in a loss of life force. This leads to an "energy-debt" in our future, in the form of a lack of vitality and a feeling of being stuck. We feel we can't move with ease on our path, since we keep dragging our past with us, and our past is now a source of wounding, toxins, and poison.

When we heal our wounds from the past, we can then bring the medicine from our healing with us into how we show up in the now. This allows us to create a future filled with this light-filled healing medicine. This is now what "shall be." In this way, the norns can help us to live our destiny, instead of our fate.

Destiny versus fate

Destiny is something you call into your life when you heal your past and start to live in alignment with your heart, soul, and spirit. You are here awake to your soul's truth, so you can tune into the whispers from your heart, guiding you to the steps you need to take in order for your highest path to unfold—your destiny.

Fate is something you end up with when you are asleep to the truth of who you are by listening to the ego's voice guiding you on your path.

We are all connected through the web of life

The concept of spirit weavers exists in many different mythologies, and I believe this is because they reveal to us a deeper truth, that we are all connected through the web of life. I have seen in my shamanic journeys, into different dimensions, how we are all part of a larger pattern, each bringing our own beautiful light and soul essence into this bigger tapestry.

Perhaps we are born with certain threads already in place, but as we make this journey of healing, awakening the Wise Woman within, we start to weave a new life into being, a life where we are being guided by our soul to the highest path available to us. And as we follow this guidance, we start to weave our soul's light and our heart's loving wisdom into our world, and by doing that we assist in birthing a new consciousness into being.

At the end of this chapter, I will take you on a shamanic journey where you will meet the Spirit Weavers from the Norse tradition, the norns, so that you can start to weave your dreams and visions into your life. Let us now meet the animal guide the Owl, who will help you to see the light in the darkness.

Owl Medicine: Seeing the Light in the Darkness

Owls are nocturnal, so they are associated with the moon. Thanks to their unique feathers, they can fly into the darkness in complete silence, and because of their amazing eyesight, they can see in near total darkness, as they are able to see even the faintest light in the dark. In this way, they are bringers of wisdom and hidden knowledge, and they can guide us through the darkness and give us signs to help us know if we are on the right path.

The Greek goddess of wisdom, Athena, has an owl sitting on her shoulder, and this owl tells Athena the truths of the world around her.

One of my animal guides is a white owl, and she helps me to see the light that is always present—in situations, in others and in myself. She can also give me very specific messages, such as when we were selling our house in Sweden to move back to the UK.

We had a house viewing, but very few prospective buyers attended. Our estate agent felt this was not a good sign, and she feared that maybe our house would be difficult to sell. This really worried me, since our daughters were due to start a new school in England a few months later and we needed to move quickly.

When the estate agent left, I went for a walk with my beautiful Bernese Mountain dog Coco. As we slowly made our way through the forest, I was deep in thought, playing out different nightmare scenarios of us being stuck in Sweden, unable to make this big move. Suddenly I heard the deep, soft sound of an owl hooting in the distance, and as I looked down on the path, I saw a white feather. I knew this was a message from my Owl.

As I came back home from my dog walk, I told my husband that I knew our house would sell. And it did! We had an offer for the asking price just a few days later, and our move went smoothly according to plan.

Our animal guides in the Spirit World can help us, by bringing us messages, just as my Owl did by giving me a reassuring message of that light-filled new path emerging in my life—a light that my physical eyes could not see. But Owl knew that our house would sell, and the feather was a sign helping me to trust that this new life was emerging, even if everything right then seemed dark.

As the Owl can see what others can't see, they help us to see our visions and dreams being sourced from the beautiful darkness of the night. They also help us to tune into our inner spiritual sight so that we can see the light that is always present, however dark the world seems.

Let us do another inquiry process, this time helping you to tune into the medicine from Owl. I recommend that you write down your answers to the following questions.

▌ Inquiry: Owl Medicine Questions

- Close your eyes, and tune into Owl. Let Owl show you all the light and goodness Owl sees in you.

- Imagine how you now fly up into the darkness of the cosmos with Owl, to the Divine Source. The first rays of the light from the sun appear in the distance and, in this emerging light, Owl now shows you a dream or a vision it wants you to become aware of. Notice what this dream or vision is.

- Owl now brings a message to you, a message that will help you on your journey through life.

I will now take you on a shamanic journey where you will meet Owl, who will share its medicine for you, helping you to see the light in the darkness. You'll then journey to the World Tree, Yggdrasil, where you'll meet the three norns, the Spirit Weavers from the Norse tradition. You will also journey to the Divine Source to receive the light of new dreams and visions.

Shamanic Journey to Meet the Spirit Weavers and Source for New Visions and Dreams

• • • • • •

Do you remember how I shared earlier about how, after my mum died, I was taken on a journey to the Land of Ice, which helped me to heal deep wounds in my psyche?

In the shamanic journey we will soon do, you will also journey to this Land of Ice, so you can discover what is frozen in your psyche. This can be from wounds held in your personal past, but also from wounds held in your ancestral lineage or in the collective.

You'll then go through a process where the ice starts to melt, allowing the life force and light that had been trapped in these frozen wounds to return to you.

In some ways, what you will experience on this part of the shamanic journey is like a soul retrieval. This is when the light-filled essence of your soul can return to you, as you heal the wounding that caused this piece of your soul to split off from you.

This disconnection from your soul's light can happen anytime you experience something that is too much for you to cope with, as your mind then suppresses the emotions and energies from that event, into your unconscious mind, where it becomes frozen. The mind does this to protect you, so you can still function. The problem with this is that you also disconnect from the life force held in your emotions, as it's now suppressed into your unconscious mind—or in shamanic terms—the lower world. This means that you lose connection with an aspect of your life force, and you can't get it back until you are willing to journey into the lower world to heal that which has become frozen.

The norn of the past, Urd, is the one who will be your guide during this process of reclaiming your life force and light, as she can help you witness that which has been frozen in your past. Urd is also an aspect of the Dark Mother, and she is so old she might even be the original ancient witch from the Norse sagas. Whoever she is for you, she is very powerful, and one of the ancient, primordial feminine forces.

You'll then meet the norn of the present, Verdandi, who will take you on a journey to the Divine Source. Here you'll receive the light-filled seeds of new dreams, visions, and inspiration. Verdandi will reveal to you how you need to show up in your life so that you can birth these dreams, visions, and inspiration into the world.

And finally, you'll meet the norn of the future, Skuld, who will reveal to you how you can weave all these dreams, visions, and inspiration into your future. It is as if she is helping to light up the highest path you are meant to take.

You can access the recording of this journey on **cissiwilliams.com/ heart**. It is 34 minutes long.

Shamanic Journey to Meet the Spirit Weavers and Source for New Visions and Dreams

Sit or lie down in a comfortable position. Close your eyes and sink into your inner stillness.

Sink deeper and deeper into the stillness, into your mystical heart, where there is a beautiful light shining, a light that is the portal that leads into the World of Spirit.

Journey through the portal into the World of Spirit

Take a deep breath in and, as you breathe out, feel how you journey through this portal into the domain of Spirit.

As you arrive in the World of Spirit, you find yourself in an ancient forest.

It is dark, the moon is shining and there is a white blanket of snow covering the ground. The frosty trees are glistening like silver in the moonlight, and the air is cold and crisp.

You notice a tree is here—your Tree of Life—and you observe how it is resting in the stillness of winter. It's like it is dreaming.

Meeting Owl

Standing here next to your tree, you suddenly hear an owl greeting you from deep within the darkness. As you look up, this beautiful owl silently comes flying toward you. The owl is one of your helpers from the Spirit World.

Allow Owl to share with you the medicine it has for you—the medicine that will help you see the light in the darkness—and any other wisdom Owl has for you.

There is a path here, in the forest, and as you keep walking on this path, you find yourself going deeper and deeper into the World of Spirit, until you come to a huge field.

In the middle of this field is a massive tree—the World Tree, Yggdrasil.

Journeying to the Well of Urd

There's an opening here by the tree, with a tunnel leading down. You start journeying down this tunnel, following the roots of the tree, going down, down, down, until you arrive at a sacred well—the well of Urd, the well of destiny.

By this well you see the three norns, who are archetypes of time, past, present, and future—three sisters who are the cosmic weavers of the web of life.

You see: the norn of the past, Urd; the norn of the present, Verdandi; and the norn of the future, Skuld.

Journey with Urd

The norn of the past, Urd, is an ancient Dark Mother, and she now steps forth, spinning a thread between her fingers. As she does this, she starts to take you on a journey to help you heal your past, so you can reclaim your life force, light and soul essence.

Feel how you journey back into the past, noticing all the old wounds where you've lost an aspect of yourself, where you've disconnected from your light and your life force.

Notice also all those parts of you that you've exiled, shut down, and locked away—wounded parts you've rejected, parts you didn't want to acknowledge.

Urd explains that all this which you've disconnected from has been frozen in your psyche, and it is now time for you to heal this.

The Land of Ice

She journeys with you, deeper and deeper into the lower world, until you come to the Land of Ice.

Here, in the Land of Ice, notice all those frozen emotions, thought patterns, memories, wounds, and rejected parts of yourself that are held deep within your psyche, all that which is frozen in your nervous system.

You may see these as metaphors, like frozen representations of those wounds, those rejected parts, those toxic emotions and old poisons that are deep below your conscious awareness, held here in this frozen Land of Ice.

Some of this may be from your own personal past, but some may be wounds from your ancestral lineage or from the collective.

Just witness it all.

Urd, who is a Dark Mother, now brings to you her holy fire of transformation.

As the fire is brought to this ice, the ice starts to melt. Let the holy fire melt all that which is frozen. Keep melting the ice.

Let it all be transformed, let all the ice melt, melt, melt, as you keep breathing out the heaviness of the past, so you also, through your breath, are releasing it into the fire.

Let it all melt.

As the ice melts it is transformed into light, into healing, so this Land of Ice transforms into a beautiful place of healing, magic, wisdom, love, and vitality.

The light returns to you

Feel how all the light that was once trapped in the ice now returns to you—all that light and life force start to return to you, from all time and space.

Let all these light-filled parts of your soul essence now come back to you—all the light that you had disconnected from when you got wounded.

Open your heart and let all this light now come back to you. Let your light come back home to you.

Healing in the Well of Urd

Urd now takes you back to her sacred well, where there is healing water flowing, the water that is the magical elixir of the divine feminine.

Urd uses this healing water to nourish the World Tree, and likewise, it can also help to nourish you, to transform you, to fill you up with light and with the life force of the feminine.

She invites you to now step inside this healing well. As you float in her holy, magical water that sparkles with light, you can feel how all the old remnants of the past are leaving you—it all flows out of your nervous system, out of your spine, out of your body, and into these holy waters, where it's being healed and transformed into light.

Let it all go—breathe it out, and let it all flow out of your body, out of your skin, and into these holy waters.

As all these remnants of the past are leaving you, feel how new space is being created within you—space that now can be filled with light, life, vitality, and energy.

Feel how you are being renewed, rejuvenated, and filled up with light, filled up with life energy from the divine feminine.

Let all this light in.

Now you step out of the well, shining so brightly, like a beautiful sun, like a radiant star, like the soft glow from the moon, from the inside out.

Journey with Verdandi

The norn of the present, Verdandi, now steps forth. She starts to spin a thread, taking you on a journey into the darkness of the sky, into the primordial womb that is the source of new light.

Feel how you start to journey up into the darkness of the sky and into a cosmic birth canal.

The birth canal opens up and you can see the shimmering light from the stars above you—a light that is like a sacred invitation, calling you to journey up to the magic found in the Divine Source of new visions and dreams.

Follow this light from the stars now, journeying up into the darkness of the cosmos, all the way up, up, up to the upper world, to the Divine Source of all that is.

As you are here now, in this magical place of divine inspiration, feel how you start to fill yourself up with all this new light that is returning to you—the light of new visions and dreams, new healing and sacred medicine.

Keep breathing in all this new light, filling you up with divine inspiration. Breathe in all this light of new life—breathe in new dreams, visions, ideas, insights, healing, and sacred medicine.

Just breathe them all in, allowing yourself to be filled up with all this light. Let this light fill you up. Let this light flow into your whole being.

Verdandi now shows you how you can show up with more wisdom and awareness in the now, so you can weave these visions and dreams, this inspiration, healing, and sacred medicine into your life.

She also shows you what she wants you to focus on in your life, so you give these new dreams and visions, inspiration, healing, and sacred medicine the time and energy they need so they can grow and blossom.

Enriched with all this light; all your insights, visions, dreams, healing, and sacred medicine, you now journey back down with Verdandi, all the way back down to the well.

Journey with Skuld

The norn of the future, Skuld, now steps forth. She is a light goddess, connecting you with your highest path, your highest choices. Skuld starts to spin a thread that takes you on a journey out into the future, where she is revealing to you how you can weave all this light, all these visions and dreams, and all these highest choices into your future—revealing to you the expansion of life that is here for you when you say YES to that which lights you up, when you say YES to be the conduit that brings all this light into the world. Then Skuld brings you back to the well.

Weaving into the web of your life

The norns now invite you to stand here with them, by the web of your life, so you can start to weave all this light of new visions and dreams and inspiration into your life.

Weave all this light and wisdom into your past.

Weave all this light and wisdom into how you show up in the now. And weave all this light and wisdom into your future, so you allow the future to blossom and unfold in the most magical way.

Feel how you are helping to birth a new consciousness into being, by weaving all this light of new visions and dreams and inspiration and healing and sacred medicine into the web of life.

Thank the three norns.

Journey back to the World Tree

And then feel how you start to journey back, journeying up the tunnel, all the way up, up, up, back to the World Tree, Yggdrasil.

As you arrive by the World Tree you see Owl here again. Take a moment now to say goodbye to Owl.

Then journey back over the field, and back onto the path that's leading through the ancient forest, to the light that is the portal in your mystical heart.

Journey back through the portal

Take a deep breath in and, as you breathe out, feel how you journey through this portal now, into your mystical heart, and back into your body.

Take another deep breath in and, as you breathe out, feel how you come back into the here and now. Take another deep breath in and, as you breathe out, you can open your eyes.

$\sim$

Write down your insights and learnings, as well as the visions and dreams and healing and sacred medicine you've just received.

If you want to, write a letter to yourself, from your heart, so it can share its messages for you.

You can start the letter with the words:

What my heart wants me to know is ...

Then put the book down and give yourself sacred time to reflect upon all the healing you have just experienced as you journeyed to meet the spirit weavers and source of new visions and dreams.

The Chamber of Magic

Flowers don't worry about how they're going to bloom.
They just open up and turn toward the light and that
makes them beautiful.

— JIM CARREY

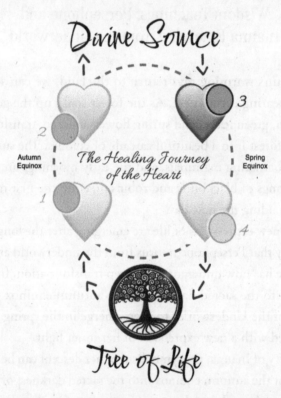

Figure 6: Entering the Third Chamber of the Heart to receive the Light

If we continue our journey following the flow of the blood, all the oxygen-rich blood now flows from the lungs and into the third chamber of the heart (number 3 in Figure 6).

This chamber represents early spring, when the Light Mothers (solar goddesses) bring the golden warm rays from the sun back to the land, nourishing the stirrings of new life.

As spring continues to approach, we journey through the portal of the spring equinox, where the darkness is left behind us, and instead we move into the magical light.

The more you allow yourself to be nourished by this light, the more you ignite the magic within you—a magic that fills your dreams and visions with the creative divine spark that expands life itself.

Wisdom Teachings: Persephone and Inanna Emerging from the Underworld

When the sun's warming rays return to the land, we can see signs of new life appearing everywhere. As the forest soaks up the golden light from the sun, green leaves and spring flowers emerge, transforming the grey winter forest into a beautiful cascade of colours. The sun's warmth wakes up hibernating mammals, and the early mornings are filled with the happy songs of blackbirds and robins greeting the first rays of light at dawn, heralding the new day.

All these new expressions of life are emerging after the long winter, in the same way that Persephone returns from the underworld at the spring equinox. She has now undergone her deep transformation, from having journeyed into the sacred darkness at the autumn equinox to become the Queen of the Underworld, to then emerge in the spring as a young maiden, filled with a new expression of her inner light.

In the story of Inanna, the symbolism of her descent can be seen as her descending at the autumn equinox into the sacred darkness of the underworld, moving through her deep transformation. She then ascends at the spring equinox, filled with a new expression of her wisdom and light.

Through these ancient myths, Persephone and Inanna illustrate the sacred cycle of birth, death, and rebirth. They reveal to us the importance of letting go, having the courage to journey into the darkness, and so moving through our own transformation. And then, with the return of the light, we emerge from the underworld, carrying within us the light of our new visions and dreams, as offerings to the world.

In this chapter, we will dive deep into how we can work with receiving the warmth and light from the returning sun, by working with the solar goddesses, so that they can help us awaken our inner magic—the magic of creation.

Let us first start with how we can receive the light to nourish our visions and dreams.

Receiving the Light to Ignite Your Inner Magic

Without the light from the sun, life would not be able to blossom and expand. It is the same with your inspirations, visions, and dreams—without them being nourished by the light, they can't grow. This means that to nourish your seeds of new life, you must be willing to *receive* this light.

But why is the sun's healing light so important?

The importance of sunlight

Sunlight is vital for the healthy functioning of our mind and body. It boosts our serotonin levels, which helps us feel happier, focused, and energized. It also strengthens our bones, rejuvenates our bodies, and reduces inflammation.

The ancient mother within you is wired into your DNA, through your maternal mitochondria. She responds to the natural cycles of darkness and light, and to the elements of earth, air, fire, and water.

She is always seeking the light, as it is this light that nourishes life. She knows that all life stems from the darkness of the womb, and she also knows that this new life must receive the light in order to grow.

Therefore, she understands how important it is for us to receive the light from the sun, from the Light Mothers, as it is the warmth and the light from the golden rays of the sun that ignites the magic of creation, allowing life to expand and blossom.

Inquiry: Questions to notice how open you are to Receiving the Light

Take a moment now to write down the answers to the questions below, so you can notice how able you are to *receive* the light from the sun. The sun is not just the actual sun in the sky, but also what it represents—love, warmth, happiness, healing, and light-filled blessings.

- Are you open to receiving warmth and love from others?
  - If yes, then that's great. If no, notice what stops you.

- How much joy do you create space for in your life?
  - If you allow for plenty of space, then that's great. If not, notice how you can free up time for that which brings you joy.

- Do you allow yourself to receive healing and support?
  - If yes, then that's wonderful. If no, notice what stops you, and how you can allow yourself to receive more support.

- Are you able to focus on the light and the blessings in your life?
  - If yes, then that's great. If no, then notice what prevents you.

- Do you say YES to that which lights you up, so you allow your life to expand and blossom?
  - If yes, then great. If no, notice what stops you.

- Do you give yourself time to regularly be outside in the sunlight?
  - If yes, then great. If no, notice if you can make time for a daily walk in the fresh air. It will boost your vitality and wellbeing.

- Do you connect with the elements of nature on a regular basis—earth, air, fire, and water?
  - If yes, then great. If no, then notice how you can weave that into your life.

- Can you walk barefoot on the earth? Can you sit regularly outside by a bonfire? Can you swim in the ocean and let the rain touch your face? Can you breathe in the fresh air outside on your daily walk?

If you notice you have an issue with receiving this light, then it is vital you heal this, which you can start to do with the shamanic journey at the end of this chapter. The more you block this light from nourishing you, the more you stop your dreams and visions from growing.

Just as the magic of creation can only blossom and expand as the buds and flowers open to receive the light from the sun, the same applies to you. Only when you allow yourself to receive nurturing light, can the magic of creation be ignited within you, so that you can blossom and expand into a new expression of life.

Therefore, trust that the more you open to receive this light, the more you strengthen your connection with the ancient mother within your bones—and SHE is the one who knows how to heal you. She is always seeking the light, so the more you connect with her, the more you receive nourishment for *you*, which ignites your inner magic.

Meet the Light Mothers Freya, Idun, and Brigid
* * * * * *

The more you allow yourself to receive the nurturing light, the more magic you develop within you, so that you can birth your dreams and visions into your life. I will here introduce you to three Light Mothers—Freya, Idun, and Brigid—who all help to ignite the magic of creation within you. You will experience their powerful medicine for you in the shamanic journey at the end of this chapter.

The Norse goddess Freya

The Norse goddess Freya is a powerful solar goddess of healing, magic, witchcraft, wisdom, love, fertility, war, and death.

She is the most powerful and formidable of the Norse goddesses, and in the Norse sagas she is described as bright, shining, wise, cunning, and very large (she is a giantess).

She is like a divine shamanic witch-priestess, and she travels the world teaching the wise women Seidr, which is a form of Norse magic, divination, and shamanic healing that was practised by *völvas* (female shamanic priestesses). She even taught Seidr to Odin, so that he could learn how to journey into the different worlds of reality. Odin was always looking to expand his knowledge of wisdom and magic from the feminine.

Freya helps you to awaken your inner magic, ancient wisdom, and healing skills, so that you can step into your feminine power and be a light in the darkness.

Freya came to me after my mum had died, as I shared in chapter two. Instead of introducing herself to me, she took me to meet the Norse dark goddess Hel, as I at that time really needed the strong healing medicine of the darkness to heal my ancestral wounds and poison.

Later, once I was further down the path of healing my deep wounding, Freya came to me again. This time she showed herself as this beautiful giantess, filled with a radiant golden light. She had long blonde hair that glowed so much that it looked as if she had a crown of light on her head.

She told me that it was time for me to receive the light from the feminine, to allow her golden healing light in. This was the next step on my healing journey.

She instructed me to visualize how I was opening up to let the light from the sun into my heart, so that the warm, golden rays could melt the ice around my heart, and heal the infection there from my inner emotional wounds. She explained that her light could heal me in the same way the sun heals us. The body heals infections and inflammations through the sun's light, and we, emotionally, feel happier through the healing properties of the sun's golden rays.

I felt how I opened my heart during every breath I took, letting Freya's golden light in. As her warm rays reached the ice around my heart,

I kept breathing out the pain that had become frozen there—and, as I did that, I could feel wave after wave of grief and sadness well up from deep within me. I kept breathing it out, allowing Freya's healing light to reach even deeper into my heart.

Freya then blew a spark of light into my heart space, igniting the divine flame in my heart. She explained that just as the sun nourishes life all around me, I was meant to let this inner fire in my heart be like a sun that could nourish the seeds of new life I was carrying within me.

She then blew a spark of light directly into my sacred womb space, my inner cauldron, and I could feel how it ignited a fire in my belly, like a fire underneath the cauldron.

She explained how my inner cauldron is the seat of my magic and that I needed to be willing to receive her golden light in order to keep the fire burning—the fire of passion, creativity, feminine power, and magic.

She then blew a spark of light into my third eye, filling it with her light. She said that it was now time for me to awaken my inner seer and see through the eyes of the Wise Woman.

That was the first time I had fully allowed the light of the feminine into me, and the peace I felt afterwards was immense. My heart felt so light, as if I had healed an old wound within me—the wound of not trusting that it was safe to receive from the feminine. As I let Freya's light in, this wound started to heal.

You will meet Freya in the shamanic journey at the end of this chapter, where she'll be igniting your inner magic too.

The Norse goddess Idun

The Norse goddess Idun is the healing soft light of the early morning sun—those first golden rays that wake up the land; so she is the bringer of dawn and spring.

Idun is the keeper of the golden apples of immortality. The seeds of these apples contain the power and magic of your life force, the essence of your light-filled soul. Even the Norse gods had to eat her apples to continue living.

These golden apples are filled with wisdom from the divine feminine, revealing to us our highest divine destiny, our highest path—so very similar to the shamanic process of destiny retrieval. These apples also help us to retrieve our life force, our light (as we do in a soul retrieval). In this way, Idun holds the essence of the light-filled life force that is weaved into all of creation.

The first time I met Idun, I was journeying to the World Tree, Yggdrasil, and I saw this beautiful goddess step out of the trunk of this tree. She had long blonde hair, that seemed to glow like gold in the sunlight. She was holding a golden apple in her hand, and she asked me to bite into it, which I did. As I kept chewing on this apple (in my inner vision), the light-filled essence from within the apple seemed to take me on a journey into the future, showing me the truth of who I am. It also revealed to me the highest path possible for me, when I said YES to that which lights me up.

You'll experience this too soon in the shamanic journey at the end of this chapter.

The Celtic goddess Brigid

The Celtic goddess Brigid is a solar goddess of spring, fertility, healing, and poetry. As she returns to the land after a long winter, the warming light from her life-giving fiery sunrays help to quicken the life that is lying dormant as seeds of potential in the cold winter earth.

Brigid is the keeper of the holy flame within your heart. She invites you to melt the ice around your heart, igniting the inner fire meant to burn so brightly within you.

She helps you to notice how you neglect your own needs, how you forget to tend to your inner fire, and her loving support helps you to amend this, so you can be filled with passion, creativity, and a zest for life.

She is also a very powerful healer, and that is how she revealed herself to me the first time I met her.

I was sitting by her holy well in Chalice Well Gardens, in Glastonbury, England, the heart chakra of the world. The spring that feeds this well is the Red Spring, which symbolizes the divine feminine. It was very early morning, and I was the only one there. The birds were singing as I sat in deep meditation by the edge of her well.

Then suddenly I felt how a presence reached up through the well, taking me on a journey into her holy waters. This happened in my inner vision, as physically I was still sitting by the edge of the well.

I realized that this presence was Brigid, and she took me on a journey back in time. First on the side of my male ancestors, on the right side of my body, where she guided me to witness, clear, release, and heal the wounding held in the masculine within me.

Wave after wave of pain and suffering caused by the insanity in the masculine surged through me and into her loving arms. It was as if she was the ancient shamanic priestess, and I was the conduit, and together we were healing aeons of ancestral and collective suffering held in the masculine.

And then it stopped, and the right side of my body felt completely empty, as if it was just a skeleton.

And then new life came in—new healthy energy of the Divine Masculine—pouring in, rebuilding the right side, as if that side of my body became a beautiful, green, strong tree, filled with life force.

Then Brigid took me on another journey, this time on the side of my female ancestors, on the left side of my body, where she guided me to witness, clear, release, and heal the wounding held in the feminine within me.

Wave after wave, the venom and the poison caused by the insanity in the feminine surged through me and into her loving arms. It was again as if she was the ancient shamanic priestess, and I was the conduit, and together we were healing aeons of ancestral and collective suffering held in the feminine.

Then it stopped, and the left side of my body felt completely empty, as if it was just a skeleton.

And then new life came in—new healthy energy of the Divine Feminine—pouring in, rebuilding the left side, as if that side of my body became a beautiful, green, strong tree, filled with flowers and blossoms.

I felt how I was being transformed into the Tree of Life, with my roots going deep down into her being, to her sacred waters, and my branches reaching high up into the heavens, to the stars and the sun and the moon.

Brigid then blew her warm breath into my heart, and I could feel how her breath carried her deep love for me, igniting the divine flame in my heart.

She whispered to me: "How can you tend to your inner divine flame in your heart, so that you allow it to continue to burn brightly?"

"How can you create more space in your life, so that your divine fire can grow even stronger?"

And then she said, "Welcome home, my child."

And I knew in that moment that I was home. I had felt so lost and disconnected, living so far away from my own ancestral land. But here, in this sacred garden at the heart chakra of the world, I had come home to the Divine Mother of the land that I was now calling home. I had connected with the Celtic solar goddess Brigid (you too will meet her soon in the shamanic journey at the end of this chapter).

All these Light Mothers—Brigid, Idun, and Freya—help you ignite your inner sun, your inner magic, so that you can use this magical light of creation to nurture your dreams and visions, until they are ready to be born through you.

You'll soon experience their medicine for you in the shamanic journey, but first let us tune into the medicine from Mama Bear so that you can open up to receive nourishment from the feminine.

Mama Bear Medicine: Receiving Nourishment from the Feminine

Mama Bear has been revered by many ancient wisdom traditions, and in Northern Europe she represented transformation and rebirth, as she journeys into the darkness of winter for her deep sleep, to emerge reborn in the spring.

The star constellation *Ursa Major* is known as The Great Bear, and it is at its lowest in the sky in autumn—as if Mama Bear is looking for a den to sleep in during her hibernation—and at its highest in the sky in the spring, when she emerges reborn.

Mama Bear is known to be a protective mother, filled with physical power, fierce courage, and strong intuition. She follows the cycle of life, death, and rebirth as she first gets pregnant in the summer, but the pregnancy will only take if she puts on enough weight in the autumn. This means that she is pregnant with new life when she enters the sacred darkness, moving into her deep sleep during her hibernation. This is when she enters the Spirit World to dream something new into being—a new dream of the life that is longing to emerge through her.

During her time in hibernation, she gives birth to her new cubs. She nurtures them, while still resting in the den, allowing them to grow stronger inside this protective space, as she knows they are not ready yet to venture out into the world. Then, as spring arrives with the returning sun, she wakes up; and, together with her cubs, emerges from their den.

In this way, Mama Bear shows us that the seeds of new life are still there, within us, even if nothing seems to be happening on the outside. As we give ourselves time to nurture these seeds of new life within us, they will eventually emerge through us, and out into the world.

But for now, we need to keep focusing on nurturing our inner "cubs"—our visions, dreams, and inspiration, so that we give them the nourishment, light, and time they need to grow.

▌ INQUIRY: Mama Bear Medicine Questions

Let us do another inquiry process, this time helping you to tune into the medicine from Mama Bear. Write down your answers to the following questions:

- How can you allow yourself to receive the nourishing light from the world around you—the blessings, love, joy, and healing—just for you?

- How can you tend to your inner fire, so that it can nourish and sustain you?

- How can you nurture your visions and dreams, so that you give them the time and space they need to grow?

I will now take you on a shamanic journey in which you'll meet Mama Bear, so she can share her medicine with you, helping you to receive the nourishing light.

You'll also meet the Light Mothers who will help to melt the ice around your heart, igniting the divine flame in your heart and your inner magic.

Shamanic Journey to Meet the Light Mothers and Ignite Your Inner Magic

In this shamanic journey, you will be filling up with the medicine from the elements—earth, air, water, and fire—connecting you with the ancient mother. You will also meet Mama Bear, and the Light Mothers.

This journey is very healing, as it opens you up to *receive the light*. And as you receive this light, you ignite the magic of creation within you, which nurtures your visions and dreams so that they can grow and expand and blossom.

I would recommend that you listen to my recording of this shamanic journey now, so that you let my voice guide you (you can access it on **cissiwilliams.com/heart**). The journey is 41 minutes long.

Shamanic Journey to Meet the Light Mothers and Ignite Your Inner Magic

Sit or lie down in a comfortable position. Close your eyes and sink into your inner stillness.

Sink deeper and deeper into the stillness, into your mystical heart, where a beautiful light is shining. This light is a portal into the World of Spirit.

Journey through the portal into the World of Spirit

Take a deep breath in and, as you breathe out, feel how you journey through this portal, into an ancient forest that is resting in the quiet stillness of winter.

Dawn is just breaking, and the gentle early morning rays of the sun are streaming through the trees, filling the forest with a magical pink, golden glow. A few birds are slowly waking up, singing softly to greet a new day.

Notice how you become a tree—the Tree of Life—with your roots going down into the earth, into the sacred darkness, filling you with nourishment, vitality, and strength.

Your branches are reaching high up, into the heavens, where they open up to receive the sun's healing rays of golden light, filling the tree with the promise of new life.

As your branches continue to receive this golden light, the tree changes from winter to early spring, with green shoots appearing on the branches.

The forest starts to transform too, with early spring flowers appearing everywhere in a cascade of vibrant colours.

You now step out of the trunk of the tree, onto a path that is leading through the forest.

You keep walking deeper and deeper into the forest until you come to a beautiful meadow.

You lie down in the soft grass, letting the earth beneath you hold you. You can hear the wind blowing through the trees and the air is filled with the fresh fragrance of the early morning dew.

Receiving the medicine

As you are lying here, let yourself begin to receive the grounding and strengthening medicine from the earth, filling you up with nourishment and healing and connection with your roots—with your ancient ancestral mother.

Let the wind blow the old cobwebs away, cleansing your

mind, so you can be filled with clarity and peace. Tune into the sacred waters of the underground rivers and wells, and from the holy dew covering the ground. Let yourself receive the healing medicine from these sacred waters of the ancient mother, so her holy waters can cleanse and rejuvenate you.

Tune into the fiery lava that is flowing like a vibrant river of life force deep within the earth. Feel how you open up to receive the medicine you need from this holy fire of the Divine Mother—a holy fire that carries her fierce love for you. Let yourself receive her love, her life force, her feminine power.

Tune into the light from the early morning sun, and open yourself up to receive her healing, golden rays that bring the promise of new life.

Just fill yourself up with that which you need.

Let yourself receive. Trust that the more you fill up with the natural elements of earth, wind, water, fire, and sunlight—the more you heal your connection with your ancient mother, the Divine Mother who is wired into your DNA.

Trust that she knows how to heal you, so let yourself receive all this light, all this healing, all this nourishing medicine for you.

Visit from Mama Bear

As you are lying here, receiving all this medicine, you notice that you are in the company of a big Mama Bear. She is sitting here next to you. She is one of your spirit helpers and she now shares with you the medicine she brings for you.

How is she meant to help you, so you can allow yourself to receive the nourishment you need?

Mama Bear stands up and she invites you now to follow her deeper into the forest. You keep following her, deeper and deeper into the forest, until you come to a large apple tree. Next to this apple tree is a little bonfire burning, a fire that's been lit just for you. A fire that represents the healing light from the sun.

Meeting Brigid and Freya

By this fire are two beautiful goddesses—one with fiery red hair, who is the Celtic goddess Brigid, and another with golden hair, who is the Norse goddess Freya.

They are here to help ignite the magic in you but, in order for your magic to flow freely, you have to melt the ice around your heart.

Feel how the heat from the fire starts to melt the ice around your heart now, so the wounding that may have frozen to ice around your heart starts to melt.

Let the warmth from the fire just melt it all away—both from in front of your heart and from behind your heart, between your shoulder blades. As you breathe out, let all the pain that was frozen within the ice be released, through your out-breath, and into the fire, where it's transformed into light.

Just keep melting the ice, releasing that which has been frozen, through your out-breath.

Healing with Brigid

Brigid now places her hands over your heart, which melts the ice even more. As the ice keeps melting, you can feel her warming up your heart, as if she is bringing it back to life.

She now blows directly into your heart space, igniting your inner divine flame. Her breath carries her love for you, so feel how you open your heart chakra to receive her love directly into your heart, igniting your inner divine flame.

Tune into this divine flame that is now burning in your heart and notice how you can tend to this inner fire, allowing it to continue to burn brightly.

How can you allow yourself to receive the light that helps to nourish this fire?

How can you create more space in your life, so your divine fire can grow even stronger?

How can you nurture your inner spark of love?

If you notice any old fears about receiving the light and expressing your love, then feel how you breathe these out, into the divine fire, so the fire can transform them all into light.

Healing with Freya

Freya now comes up to you. She places her hands over your sacred womb space, releasing from you all that may have blocked you from stepping into your creative power, magic, and light.

Just let it all go. Release it as you breathe out into this holy fire. Let it all be released into the holy fire, all your old fears of being the Wise Woman that you are—a Wise Woman filled with feminine magic. Let it all be released into the fire where it is transformed into light.

Freya now releases from your throat all those old blocks and fears about expressing your power, being in your power, and sharing your light and magic with the world.

Just be willing to let it all go—all these old fears that blocked you from speaking your soul's truth—and place it all in the holy fire.

Feel how all these old fears and wounded energy pours out of your throat and into the fire. Just let it pour out of your throat, releasing it for every out-breath, and see and feel and trust how the fire transforms it into light.

Freya now removes from your third eye that which may have blocked your spiritual sight—releasing old blocks, fears, and programming from your past—placing it all in the holy fire, where the fire transforms it into light.

Freya now fills you up with her golden healing light, so you start to glow and radiate from this golden light. She pours this golden healing light into your sacred womb space, into your heart, into your throat, and into your third eye.

Just keep receiving all this healing light from her. As you open up to receive her light directly into your womb, heart, throat, and third eye, feel how the old fears, blocks, and wounded energy melt away. It is as if her healing golden light starts a deep detox within you, like a purging, where all this old, wounded energy and toxins start to pour out of your skin, your eyes, your hair, your hands, and your feet.

Let it all be released from deep within, as you continue to open up to receive the golden healing light from Freya directly into your womb, heart, throat, and third eye.

Let yourself receive her healing light.

Let it in, let it in, let it in, and allow all that which is not in alignment to be released from you until you are glowing with light.

Freya now blows her light directly into your sacred womb space, into your inner cauldron, filling it with her creative power, with her magic—the feminine magic of the Wise Woman.

Tune into this magic that is now brewing in your inner cauldron and let this magic reveal to you how you can step into your feminine power in your life.

Freya now blows her light directly into your heart, filling your heart with her fierce compassion and loving wisdom—the fierce compassion and wisdom of the Wise Woman.

Tune into your heart and ask your fierce compassion what it wants you to know, so you can allow this fierce love to guide you on your path.

Freya now blows her light directly into your throat chakra, filling it with the courage to speak your soul's truth.

Tune into your throat chakra and notice how you can give voice to the Wise Woman within you, so you can share her magical power and wisdom with others.

Freya now blows her light directly into your third eye, filling you up with divine sight, awakening your inner seer, so you can see through the eyes of the Wise Woman.

Tune into these eyes of the Wise Woman and let them reveal to you what you are now willing to see, as you look through her eyes—the eyes of the Wise Woman.

Meeting Idun

The trunk of the apple tree now opens up, and the Norse goddess Idun steps forth. Her blonde hair is glowing like the sun.

She is holding a shining golden apple in her hand. This apple is filled with the light and essence of your soul's highest path, your highest potential, and your highest wisdom.

Idun invites you to bite into this apple. As you take a bite, and you start to chew, the light-filled essence from the golden apple starts to reveal to you the truth of who you are.

As you keep chewing this golden light-filled apple, Idun takes you on a journey, revealing to you your highest choices, your highest path. She shows you how you can choose to say YES to that which lights you up, as this light will guide you to the path that is meant for you. Idun now brings you back to the apple tree.

Being nourished by the golden light

Freya, Brigid and Idun start to fill you with their golden light. Feel how this light flows into your crown chakra, your third eye, your throat chakra, your heart chakra, your solar plexus, your womb space, and your root chakra.

Let this golden light nurture you. Allow yourself to open up and receive all this golden healing light.

The more you let this golden light nurture you, the more it ignites the sun that shines in your heart. And as this sun in your heart starts to glow and radiate, it nurtures the visions, dreams, inspiration, and soul gifts that you are carrying within you, so they can grow and blossom.

Just like Mama Bear nourishes her young, you too need to nourish your soul gifts and dreams. And just like Mama Bear allows herself to be nourished by the Great Mother, you too need to allow yourself to receive nourishment from the Light Mothers.

The more light you receive, the more you can nurture your soul gifts and dreams—so they can later emerge into the world.

So let yourself receive all this golden healing light, and let your inner sun glow, glow, glow, filling your soul gifts and dreams with the spark of life, with the magic of creation.

Keep breathing in this light. Keep opening yourself up to receive this light, strengthening the glowing rays of the sun in your heart, filling your inner cauldron with magic, and filling your third eye with so much light that you can see through the eyes of the Wise Woman, you can witness the magic of life all around you.

Now it's time to journey back, so say goodbye to Mama Bear, Freya, Idun, and Brigid. As you start walking back on the path that is leading through the forest, you are glowing and radiating like a sun, brightening up the forest around you.

Becoming the Tree of Life

Journey all the way back to your Tree of Life. Feel how you step inside this tree—with your roots going deep down into the earth, being nourished by the medicine from the sacred darkness. Let these roots grow stronger and stronger, deepening your connection with Mother Earth.

Your branches reach high up into the sky, and the leaves are opening up even more than before, so they can soak up all the healing and magical light from the sun. Your branches are filled with beautiful blossoms, spreading their divine fragrance in the air.

Your heart is still shining like a sun in your chest—filling you with vitality, happiness, love, and the magic of life itself. Just like the sun nourishes all of life around you, you are meant to let your inner sun nourish the seeds of new visions and dreams and feminine magic you carry within you.

Trust that the feminine wisdom within you knows how to birth all these seeds of new life, visions, and dreams, at the right divine timing. All you have to do, right now, is to keep receiving the light, so all your seeds of new life can be nourished and filled with the magic of creation.

177

Journey back through the portal

Take a deep breath in and, as you breathe out, feel how you tune into the portal that leads into your mystical heart.

Take another deep breath in and, as you breathe out, bring all this light, all this magic, all this wisdom, all this nourishment, all these insights and messages from the World of Spirit with you—back into your body, and back into the here and now.

Take another deep breath in and, as you breathe out, you can open your eyes.

～

Take a few moments now to write down your insights and learnings.

If you want to, write a letter to yourself, from your heart, and perhaps also from the Light Mothers so that they can share with you their messages for you.

You can start the letter with the words:

What my heart and the Light Mothers want me to know is ...

Then put the book down and give yourself sacred time to reflect upon all the healing you have just experienced.

The Chamber of Rebirth

*A heart filled with love is like a phoenix that
no cage can imprison.*

— RUMI

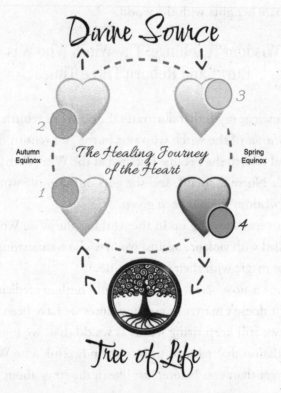

Figure 7: Entering the Fourth Chamber of Rebirth

If we continue our journey, following the flow of the blood, then all the oxygen-rich blood has now moved from the third chamber, through the heart valve (which represents the portal of the spring equinox, as can be seen in Figure 7), and into the fourth chamber.

This chamber is another powerhouse in the heart (second and fourth chambers are the bigger ones), as this is the chamber that pumps all the oxygen-rich blood out into the whole body, so the body can be nourished and filled with the life of spirit.

The medicine of the fourth chamber is to move us through our own rebirth, where we emerge with a new expression of our light, ready to share our soul gifts, healing medicine, visions, and dreams with others.

This chamber represents what Mother Earth does in early summer, when she has moved through her own rebirth, allowing life to blossom, so she can share her gifts with the world.

Wisdom Teachings: The Witch Who Was Burnt and Reborn Three Times

• • • • • •

A beautiful ancient myth that illustrates the power of rebirth is the story from the *Völuspá* of the witch who was burnt and reborn three times. After her final rebirth she became initiated as the Wise Woman, the First Völva (female Norse shaman), and she goes out into the world, sharing the magical wisdom she has been given.

Many of us fear showing up in the world as the Wise Woman, since our past is filled with violence against women who were sharing their light and feminine magic with their communities.

But the time is now here for us to share our healing medicine with the world. And it doesn't matter how many times we have been suppressed in the past, we still keep rising. And, as we do that, we move through our own initiation that rebirths us into the powerful Wise Woman that we are, stronger than ever before, just like in the story about Gullveigr.

The witch who was three-times burnt and three-times born

Gullveigr appears in the *Völuspá* (the prophecy of the witch), where she is being burnt and stabbed three times by the Norse sky gods—who represent the masculine and the mind—but each time she is reborn. After the last rebirth, she becomes the First Völva. She then goes out into the world sharing her Seidr teachings (Norse shamanism and magic), especially with "wicked" women who all loved her (and the word "wicked" comes from wicca, which means "wise," so she is teaching the wise women).

It is the goddess Freya who appears as Gullveigr in the *Völuspá*, so she is the First Völva.

Freya is here demonstrating that she has the power to resurrect and rebirth herself, something the Norse gods could not do—as they had to eat of Idun's apples—so her feminine magic is very powerful.

According to the Norse scholar Maria Kvilhaug, the name *Gullveigr* means a "gold power drink," where the gold is a metaphor for something deeply mysterious—the light found in magic, divine power, and sacred knowledge. It is the golden light of our eternal soul. In the Norse sagas, the soul is feminine, while the mind is masculine.

This golden drink represents "mead," which is the precious drink only given by the goddess—a golden drink that provides sacred wisdom and resurrection from death.

Gullveigr is the one that is the source of this golden drink, just as Freya is the source of Seidr, healing, magic, and witchcraft.

Maria Kvilhaug shares in her book *The Seed of Yggdrasil* that this myth is a story of initiation, where Gullveigr gets burnt and stabbed three times, moving through her own symbolic death and resurrection—like Inanna did. As Gullveigr passes this test of initiation, she takes on a new name, Heiðr, which means "bright one," so she has now become illuminated. Then she goes out into the world teaching the wise women about Seidr.

In this way, the story about Gullveigr is illustrating how we must be willing to undergo our own initiation in order to awaken the Wise Woman within—the one that holds our ancient feminine magic and power.

In the shamanic journey at the end of this chapter you will go through your own initiation where you'll burn and rise from the ashes three times, so that the Wise Woman within you can be reborn.

But let us first look at how you can release the deep fears that stop you from being the light that you are, sharing your soul gifts with the world.

Releasing What Stops You from Receiving the Light So That You Can Move Through Your Own Rebirth

Many of us have deep fears that hinder us from receiving the light needed to ignite our inner magic so that we can move through our own rebirth, where we emerge ready to share our visions and dreams and be the light that we are in the world. This is why it is vital to look at what fears may be blocking us.

What fears can stop you from receiving the light?

There are many layers of fears that can stop us from receiving the light, such as:

- The need to always be busy, by focusing on thinking, doing, and taking action. This can effectively stop us from being able to be still, and it is in this stillness that the light of Spirit can come to us, in the form of a flash of new insight, guidance, knowing or vision.

- The inability to be comfortable in the stillness, waiting for something new to be born. Until we embrace the stillness, and the "not-knowing," the mind will freak out, trying to analyse and forcefully find a path forward. But when we allow ourselves to drop into the stillness, a light will gently appear that guides us to the next step. And, as we follow that next step, the path unfolds.

- Feeling unworthy of receiving the light is very common. This occurs when we somehow believe we are bad, so we block ourselves from receiving that which we know is good for us, depriving ourselves of the healing medicine found in the light. When we do this, we deny our inner visions and dreams the nourishment they need to be born into the world.

- Fears about receiving the nourishing light from the feminine, due to deep wounds of not feeling safe with the feminine. This causes us to block ourselves from receiving the light that we need to grow, and instead we try to do it all on our own. But just as a cancer cell thinks it knows better than the Divine Intelligence that runs the body—which is kind of insane—it won't work for us either in the long run. Instead, when we tune into the Divine Mother who creates life itself, we move in sync with her wisdom, and this allows life to expand and blossom through us. Trusting that the Divine Mother loves us, helps us to open to receive her nourishing light.

In the shamanic journey at the end of this chapter, you'll be releasing some of these fears that may have stopped you from *receiving* the light and, as they are released, you start to move through your own rebirth.

But before we go on this journey, let us now also look at the fears you may have about *rising* from the ashes reborn.

Rising from the Ashes Reborn

We can see in the story about Gullveigr the importance of letting our old self die, by having the courage to step into the fire of renewal, so that we can be reborn into something new.

But although we can logically see the beautiful symbolism of this, the reality is that often we have deep fears about stepping into the power and magic held in the feminine. And these fears can effectively stop us from daring to step into that cosmic fire that we know will burn us down to the ground, as we might fear what will happen to us when we rise from the ashes reborn. Will we be shunned and exiled from our friendships? Will we be persecuted and vilified? Will we be considered weird and somehow bad?

These are all valid fears, given past soul experiences of being persecuted, vilified, shunned, and exiled. But as we let those old fears burn down to the ground, we are liberated from the chains of the past so that we can move through this rebirth, and go out there and share our healing medicine and loving wisdom with our family, friends, communities, and the world.

There is a beautiful connection between the Scorpion, Eagle, and Phoenix that illustrates this journey of releasing our fears and having the courage to move through our transformation and rebirth.

The Scorpion, Eagle, and Phoenix

The ancient Egyptians honoured the Scorpion as they viewed it as a being of the underworld, representing the process of death, transformation, and rebirth.

The month of Scorpio is in the dark months of early winter, which is when we enter the Dark Mother's underworld (symbolized by the medicine of the second chamber of the heart).

This is the stage of Scorpio, where we start to look at all the ways in which we get caught in our deeper wounds, and how we unconsciously may sting other people with our venom when we are triggered by these wounds. As we start to heal these deep wounds, we move through a transformation, where we enter the stage of Eagle.

As the Eagle, we can now fly more freely above the turmoil of the world, while still being able to witness what is going on down there on the ground. We have more wisdom and clarity available to us. Here, we start to look at whether we serve just ourselves, or the whole.

As we choose to serve the whole, we move through a third transformation, entering the stage of the Phoenix. This is when we are reborn from the ashes, resurrected into our light, into our divine power, where we recognize that we are here to serve a greater power than our own. We are here to serve the whole.

This is the stage where the Scorpion has broken free from the chains of the past, and instead surrendered to being guided by love. In so doing, it gets its spiritual wings as the Phoenix, so that it can fly out into the world and serve others.

This is the medicine of the fourth chamber—to move through this rebirth, where you get your spiritual wings so that you can serve others, by sharing your soul gifts and healing medicine.

To reach this stage of serving others, we must be willing to heal our fears in relation to rising from the ashes reborn, so let us look at what some of these may be for you. As you later release these fears in the shamanic journey at the end of this chapter, you'll move through these three stages of the Scorpion, Eagle, and Phoenix.

Three inquiry steps to discover your fears of rising from the ashes reborn

Many layers of fears can block us from daring to step into the fire of transformation and rebirth. To help you discover what some of these fears may be for you, answer the following questions on paper.

Fears about the Circle of Sisterhood:

Notice the fears you have from having been attacked, vilified, blamed, and stung by the venom of other women. Also notice how you have attacked, vilified, blamed, and stung them. As you heal this, you move through the stage of Scorpion.

Fears about the Circle of Wise Women:

Notice the deep wounds you carry in relation to the persecution, suppression, and vilification of the wise women. Deep wounds that may have caused you to hide your power and magic, wounds that caused you to fall asleep to who you truly are. Wounds that stopped you from being able to see the wisdom and clarity available to you. As you heal this, you move through the stage of Eagle.

Fears about the Sacred Circle of Ancient Wise Witches:

Notice the fears you have about the ancient wise witches who existed before time—the dark feminine primordial forces. Notice how the old patriarchal programming caused you to fear them, which stopped you from accessing their love, power, and magic for you. Also notice how this fear stopped you from daring to be of service to the world, as the Wise Woman you are. As you heal this, you move through the transformation, becoming like the Phoenix rising from the ashes reborn.

We will soon do a very powerful journey in which you release these deep fears, but before we do that, let's discover in more depth the medicine from Eagle and Phoenix.

Eagle and Phoenix Medicine: Follow What Lights You Up

• • • • • •

The Eagle and Phoenix, both powerful animal allies in the Spirit World, look similar but carry slightly different medicines that can help you.

Eagle Medicine

The Eagle helps you to soar, high up in the sky, wing to wing with Spirit, with clear, focused vision. Eagle medicine can help you to see the bigger picture by flying above the tiny details of life, but it also shows you that once it decides on something that it can swoop down and take what it needs with incredible speed and precision.

Eagle helps you to tune into Spirit, so that you can hear, feel, see, and know the guidance from the Divine.

Eagle is connected with the rising sun, so it is helping you to follow the light of what is rising in your life, to say YES to that which lights you up. It whispers to you that it is time now to fly into the light, trusting that this light is good, right, and beautiful.

Phoenix Medicine

The Phoenix resembles an eagle, but with beautiful rich red and gold colours. It represents rebirth and resurrection, as at the end of its life it sets itself on fire, letting the fire burn through it until it dies. And then, from the ashes, a new Phoenix rises.

It shows us that we can move through our own transformation, to be reborn from the ashes of the old, just as Gullveigr was reborn as the First Völva, when the sky gods tried to burn her three times.

Phoenix whispers to you that you have all this magic, light, and feminine wisdom within you, and that it is time for you now to let her RISE.

Let us do another inquiry process, this time helping you to tune into the medicine from Eagle and Phoenix.

▌ INQUIRY: Eagle Medicine Questions

- Close your eyes and imagine you soar high above your life.
- What is the bigger vision Eagle has for your life?
- As you look out at the horizon, seeing the rising sun, notice the light that is rising in your life.
- Which areas of your life are shining from this emerging light?
- Observe what activities, relationships, and life areas light you up.
- How can you give yourself more time, energy, and focus to follow that which lights you up?

▌ INQUIRY: Phoenix Medicine Questions

- What is meant to be released so that it can be transformed in the Cosmic Fire?
- This could be old ideas, identities, or situations.
- What is longing to rise from the ashes, so that it can be reborn through you?
- What is the magic that is brewing within you, which you are meant to share as you dare to move through your own initiation into the Wise Woman?

Let us now do a shamanic journey together where you meet Eagle and Phoenix. You'll also move through your own resurrection and rebirth, where you grow huge spiritual wings so that you can fly out into the world sharing your soul gifts and healing medicine with others.

Shamanic Journey of Initiation: The Wise Woman Rising from the Ashes Reborn

In this shamanic journey, you will meet Eagle and Phoenix, who will take you on a journey where you'll release the fears that block you from being the light that you are. You'll also move through a deep initiation, being burnt three times to the ground. Each time rising, reborn into the truth of who you are.

At the end of the journey, you'll meet the ancestral witch in your lineage, the Wise One, who will share her medicine and wisdom with you. I strongly recommend that you go on this journey when you are filled with energy, as it is quite long and VERY powerful (it is 50 minutes long). You can access the recording of my voice guiding you through this shamanic journey on **cissiwilliams.com/heart.**

Shamanic Journey of Initiation: The Wise Woman Rising from the Ashes Reborn

Close your eyes and sink into your inner stillness. Into your mystical heart, where there's a beautiful light shining. A light that is a portal into the World of Spirit.

Journey through the portal

Take a deep breath in and, as you breathe out, feel how you journey through this portal now, into an ancient forest.

It's early morning, with the first morning rays from the sun streaming through the treetops, creating a magical golden glow that fills the whole forest. The birds are singing softly, welcoming you to this sacred place.

You notice how you are becoming a tree—the Tree of Life—with your roots going down into the sacred darkness of the earth, and the branches going up, into the magical light from the heavens.

The tree starts to change appearance, moving from spring to early summer, with blossoms appearing on the branches, filling the air with their beautiful fragrance.

The trunk of the tree opens up, and you step out.

Walking on the path through the forest

You notice there is a path in front of you, a path that is leading through this forest. You start walking on this path, taking you deeper into the forest, inhaling the scents of the damp moss underneath your feet, the sweet fragrance from wildflowers covering the ground, and the freshness of the dew covering the bushes and plants.

You keep walking deeper and deeper into the forest until you come to a clearing, where there is a bonfire burning.

Meeting Eagle and Phoenix

Next to the fire, you see Eagle and Phoenix. They are here to guide you on this journey of rebirth.

Tune into Eagle now, and let Eagle share its medicine with you—revealing the bigger vision for your life, how you can follow what lights you up, and how you can choose to witness the light that is rising in your life.

Tune into Phoenix now, and let Phoenix share its medicine with you—revealing what you are meant to let go of in the cosmic fire of renewal that's burning here, so you can be transformed and rise from the ashes reborn.

It's time for you now to release into the fire everything you are meant to let go of so it can be transformed.

Feel how you breathe into the fire all the ways in which you block yourself from receiving the light—perhaps you keep yourself so busy you can't receive it, or you avoid being still?

Or your mind keeps hunting for solutions, constantly trying to solve everything, not trusting the wisdom found in the stillness of the feminine.

Notice what is blocking you from receiving the light from the feminine and place it all in the fire.

Place in the fire now all the ways in which you block yourself from being nourished by the light—perhaps you feel unworthy of it, or you somehow fear receiving the life-giving light from the feminine?

Place whatever you notice is blocking you from being nourished by this magical, feminine light into the fire.

Eagle and Phoenix explain to you that you are going on a sacred journey where you'll burn down to the ground three times—each time you will rise and be reborn into the truth of who you are.

They start flying ahead of you, guiding you deeper into the forest, until you arrive at another bonfire. Around this fire, you see a sacred circle of sisters.

Healing the wounds in the circle of sisters

These sisters now share with you the wounds you carry from the circle of sisterhood—the wounds from having been attacked, judged, blamed, and stung by the venom from your sisters; and the wounds from you having attacked, judged, blamed, and stung them, and yourself.

Feel those wounds in your body, in your psyche, and in your consciousness now.

Feel the infection from those wounds held in the sacred circle of sisters for you—the wounds that caused the circle to break for you.

Feel the venom.

Trust that you are here now, by this fire, to heal it.

Step inside this divine fire now, trusting its healing and transformative powers—and, as you are inside this healing, cleansing, divine fire, let it all burn, burn, burn.

Feel how you are being released from these deep wounds held

in your body, in your psyche, in your nervous system, in your heart, in your ancestral lineage, and in your roots—let the fire burn through you.

Feel how all the old wounds, old infections, old poisons, and venom are being burnt in this divine fire—freeing your spine, freeing your heart, freeing your roots, freeing your hands and feet, freeing your eyes and ears and hair, freeing your body and thoughts, freeing your consciousness—freeing your whole being.

Just let it all go. Breathe it out, scream it out, stomp it out. Let it all burn, burn, burn. Let yourself be healed. Let yourself be freed.

Feel yourself burn, burn, burn—down to the ground—until you are just ashes, and the past no longer has a hold on you.

And now you rise, rise, rise, reborn—into the truth of who you are, when you are embodying the loving wisdom of the sacred sisterhood. So just rise, rise, rise. Feel how you expand and blossom into this new expression of the loving truth of who you are.

Eagle and Phoenix now continue to guide you onto the path, leading you deeper and deeper into the forest, until you arrive at another bonfire.

Healing the wounds in relation to the Wise Women

Around this holy fire, you see a sacred circle of Wise Women. They share with you the wounds you carry in relation to the persecution, suppression, and vilification of the Wise Women— deep wounds that caused you to hide your power and your magic, wounds that caused you to fall asleep to who you truly are. In this sleep, you forgot the wisdom, clarity, and ancient truth that was always available to you.

Feel these wounds in your body, in your psyche, in your consciousness now.

Feel what these wounds have done to this sacred circle of Wise Women—feel how this has affected you. Trust that you are here now, by this fire, to heal it.

Now step inside this holy transformative fire, and let all those wounds of persecution, of suppression, of violence and insanity for being the Wise Woman that you are, now come up within you, and let them all burn, burn, burn in this holy fire.

Let it all burn, burn, burn—scream it out, vomit it out, stomp it out, shake it out—feel the fire of holy rage burn, burn, burn through you—feel yourself screaming "NO MORE!!!!!"

Let this holy fire burn, burn, burn through you—releasing you from the insanity, the bondages from the past—the chains, the ropes, the old ways of keeping you bound; let it all burn, burn, burn.

Let it all burn, burn, burn—down to the ground—until you are just ashes, and these old fears, these old wounds, no longer have a hold on you.

And then you rise, you rise, you rise, reborn—into the truth of who you are—that you are a Wise Woman, here to take your place in the sacred circle of Wise Women. A Wise Woman who can see through the eyes of wisdom and clarity.

Eagle and Phoenix now continue to guide you on to the path, leading you deeper into the forest, until you arrive at another bonfire.

Healing the wounds in relation to the ancient witches

Around this fire, you see a sacred circle of ancient witches, ancient wise ones, who were here before time itself.

These ancient wise witches now share with you all those old beliefs, fears, and programming that caused you to fear them, to deny them, or to make them into something that they are not, which stopped you from being able to access their power, their magic, and their love *for you*. They are the primordial feminine forces that helped to birth our world—and they love you!

Feel all those wounds that you carry in your body, in your psyche, in your heart, and in your consciousness from having feared these loving, ancient, primordial feminine forces—these ancient wise witches that existed before time itself.

Feel what these wounds have done to you, how they have caused you to disconnect from your own source, from your own power, your own magic.

Trust that you are here now, by this holy fire, to heal it all.

Step inside this holy fire now, with these ancient wise witches as your witnesses. Let all these old fears come up within you, all the ways in which you have blocked yourself from connecting with your power, with your magic, with the ancient witch that lives inside of you.

Let all the fears that have caused you to be chained and gagged for thousands of years now come up within you—and let all these old fears, wounds, and old patriarchal programming burn, burn, burn.

Let it all burn, burn, burn. Breathe it out, scream it out, stomp it out, shake it out, vomit it out—let it all be released.

Let it all burn, burn, burn—down to the ground—until you are just ashes and these old fears and programming no longer have a hold on you.

And now you rise, you rise, you rise—reborn into the ancient truth that you are LOVE itself. You are an embodiment of the wisdom, light, magic, and power of the ancient wise witch, the witch-within-wood—the witch within the core of your being.

Now step out of the fire, as an embodiment of this ancient wisdom that you are, an ancient wisdom that is here to serve the world.

The ancient witches around the fire smile and welcome you back into the sacred circle of this ancient divine feminine wisdom that is yours.

Welcoming the light back

Now as you have risen and been reborn three times—all the light and magic that you previously had disconnected from starts returning to you, from all time and space. Open your heart and soul and welcome all this light and magic back to you now.

Feel how you start to glow and radiate with light, as you welcome back all this light and magic that is now returning to you.

Open up even more and welcome back all the light-filled parts that are now returning to you, with gifts of healing, power, and magic from the Wise Woman that you are, through all time and space—from the sacred circle of Wise Women.

Open up and welcome back all the light-filled parts that are now returning to you, with gifts of trust, joy, friendship, and love from the sacred circle of sisters. Feel how you glow and radiate with all this light.

Meeting the Ancient Witch from your ancestral lineage

As the light that you are, you are now ready to meet her, the ancient one, the Ancient Witch from your ancestral lineage—the one who births all life, who births the light, who is the ancient original source of your power and magic and wisdom.

Eagle and Phoenix guide you to a hidden opening in the ground. It is dark inside, and you keep walking deeper and deeper into the darkness, deeper and deeper, until you come to a holy well, filled with the dark holy waters of the Dark Mother.

On the other side of the well, you see HER—the ancient wise one, the ancient ancestral witch who is here for *you*.

She is connected with you, through your blood, your bones, your roots.

She is here to give you messages, and to share with you her healing medicine, wisdom, magic, and feminine power that will help you on your journey through life. Notice what it is she wants to share with you now.

What are the soul gifts you are meant to bring into the world, what is the magic you are meant to share with others, what is the ancient divine feminine power you are meant to embody, so you help to share the healing medicine from the Wise Woman with the world?

The ancient wise one now gives you a gift, a healing medicine she wants you to bring through into your life, into our world, from her. Notice what it is, and how you are meant to share it.

Then thank her and say goodbye.

Back to the circle of ancient witches

Eagle and Phoenix now lead you out of this holy place, back to the circle of the ancient witches, where you now share with them the medicine and gifts you've just been given, from the ancient wise one, the ancient witch of your ancestral lineage.

These ancient witches now give you their gifts for you that will help you on your journey. Notice what these gifts are, and how you are meant to use them.

Back to the circle of Wise Women

Enriched with all your gifts, Eagle and Phoenix guide you back to the path that takes you to the circle of Wise Women, where you now share with them all the medicine and gifts you've just been given from the ancient witches, and from the loving, ancient wise one.

The Wise Women now give you their gifts for you, gifts that will help you on your journey. Notice what these gifts are, and how you are meant to use them.

Back to the circle of sisters

Enriched with all these gifts, Eagle and Phoenix guide you back to the path that takes you to the sacred circle of sisters, where you now share with them all the medicine and gifts you've just been given from the ancient wise one, the ancient witches and the Wise Women.

The sisters that are here for you, in this sacred circle of sisterhood, now give you their gifts for you, gifts that will help you on your journey. Notice what these gifts are, and how you are meant to use them.

Enriched with all these gifts from the ancient wise witch of your ancestral lineage, the ancient witches, the Wise Women, and the sacred circle of sisters, Eagle and Phoenix now lead you back to the path in the forest.

Back to the path in the forest

Feel how the golden light from the sun is filling you with magic, with the healing life-giving rays from the sun.

Feel how the soft silvery light from the moon is filling you with intuition and wisdom.

Growing your spiritual wings

Feel how your heart opens as you receive all this medicine from the darkness and the light. As your heart opens, you start to grow your spiritual wings. Notice how your left wing is connecting you with the moon, with the Dark Mothers, with the power, transformation, and healing medicine of the sacred darkness, with the guiding light from the moon, and the shimmering stars at night.

The other wing, your right wing, is connecting you with the sun, with the Light Mothers, with the medicine from the light that gives life, with the golden healing rays from the sun that heal your body, soothe your soul, and ignite the divine flame in your heart. The light that nourishes and sustains you and gives you the light-filled seeds of new visions, dreams, ideas, insights, and inspiration.

You need both wings in order to fly—your left wing connecting you with the medicine of the sacred darkness, and your right wing connecting you with the medicine of the magical light.

Notice how your spiritual wings grow bigger and bigger and bigger and, as you stretch them out, see how big they are ... and then, you take off, letting your spiritual wings carry you high, high, high—up, up, up, into the sky—flying above the world, filling your life with the medicine from the magical light and the sacred darkness, and with all the wisdom you've received from the World of Spirit.

Fill your life with all your insights and visions and dreams and soul gifts and healing medicine—just sprinkle all of this into your life.

As you are flying up here, over the world, filling it with light, healing, and wisdom, ask the Divine Mothers of Darkness and Light: "How may I serve?"

Listen to their answers.

Start to fly back to the path in the forest, bringing all your wisdom, insight, gifts, and healing medicine with you.

Thank Eagle and Phoenix for being here with you, as your spirit allies, and thank the Divine Mothers of Darkness and Light.

Let us now prepare to journey back. Feel how you start to journey back to the path in the forest, and back to the portal that leads into your mystical heart.

Journey back through the portal

Take a deep breath in and, as you breathe out, feel how you journey through this portal, bringing with you your spiritual wings—one connecting you with the Dark Mothers, the other connecting you with the Light Mothers—all the way back into your mystical heart, back into your body, and back into the here and now.

Take another deep breath in and, as you breathe out feel how you bring all this light and wisdom through, into your physical reality, into your relationships, into your activities, into your life here. Just keep breathing all this light, healing, and wisdom into the areas of your life that need them the most.

Keep doing this at your own pace.

Take another deep breath in and, as you breathe out, you can open your eyes.

⌒

Take a few moments now to write down your insights and learnings. If you want to, write a letter to yourself, from your heart, and perhaps also from the Wise Woman within, so that they can share with you their messages for you.

You can start the letter with the words:

*What my heart and my inner Wise Woman want me
to know is ...*

Then put the book down and give yourself sacred time to reflect upon all the healing you have just experienced.

Part 3

Weaving Your Heart's Wisdom into Your World

Re-Writing Your Story

Your heart is not a fragile, delicate bird, but a resilient,
powerful hawk learning to fly.
— HEATHERASH AMARA

Your heart has now taken you through an intense journey of healing, transformation, magic, and rebirth, where you have awakened the Wise Woman within, so that you can share your soul gifts and healing medicine with those you meet.

As you prepare to bring all of this into your life, it is vital that you continue to see through the eye of the heart, trusting its infinite wisdom and loving guidance, while letting go of the need for external validation.

In this same way, Mary Magdalene had to trust the spiritual eye of her heart when she witnessed Yeshua after he had risen. Yeshua is the Aramaic name for Jesus, the language spoken at that time. Despite no one else being able to back up the validity of what she had experienced, she still shared her soul gifts and healing medicine with others—the gift of her faith, and the healing medicine of her courage—so that she could weave her heart's loving wisdom into our world.

I feel there are so many correlations between how Mary Magdalene's voice was silenced and intentionally distorted by patriarchy for more than 1500 years, and how the feminine has been silenced and intentionally distorted for millennia.

And just as the ancient feminine within us now is rising, the ancient teachings of Mary Magdalene are also rising in our collective consciousness, giving us the courage to share our heart's wisdom, so that we can weave it into our lives. But who was Mary Magdalene, and how can her wisdom teachings help us now?

The Ancient Wisdom Teaching of Mary Magdalene Is Rising Again

• • • • • •

All the four gospels in the New Testament recognize that Mary Magdalene was there, during the crucifixion of Yeshua, and that she was the one to first have a vision of him. This means that she is instrumental in the teachings of Christ, as she is the one to tell the good news that he had risen.

But although she is fundamental to the birthing of Christianity, she seems to completely disappear from the Bible, as if her importance was pushed underground.

Rewriting Her-Story

After Yeshua's crucifixion and resurrection, many texts appeared outlining his teachings, but only those that fit a patriarchal narrative were later included in the New Testament, around the end of the fourth century.

Scholar Karen L. King, professor of Divinity at Harvard University, refers to this as the "Master Story," where only the gospels that could guarantee the uniformity of Christian belief and practice (where men were in power) were included in the New Testament. All the other early Christian gospels were declared heresy, to establish these more orthodox gospels.

The early church fathers had a few concerns with Mary Magdalene's presence in Yeshua's life—for example, that Yeshua had appeared to her first and instructed her to tell the others, meaning that a woman could teach men.

They were also concerned that Yeshua had told her not to touch him when she had her initial vision of him, as this could be seen as proof that his resurrection was spiritual, and not physical.

Despite these concerns, they initially viewed her through positive eyes.

Then something happened, and Karen L. King explains this with such clarity in her book the *Gospel of Mary of Magdala*.

She reveals how, from the fourth century onward, the tone changed, so much so that Yeshua's comment to Mary Magdalene—that she could not touch him when she had her vision of him—was now viewed as a sign that she was unworthy of touching the risen Christ, as she lacked full understanding of the resurrection, and therefore she was weak in her faith. This was the reason, it was argued, that she was sent to tell the other disciples, so that her perceived weakness could be supplemented by the men's strength.

Then, in A.D. 591, the story around Mary Magdalene became even more distorted, when Pope Gregory I declared that Mary Magdalene was the unnamed sinner woman anointing Yeshua's feet. He also stated that her greatest sin was lust, and that the seven demons cast out of Mary Magdalene were the seven deadly sins.

Nothing in the older scriptures had supported this sudden assumption. Episcopal priest and mystic Cynthia Bourgeault, writes in her book *The Meaning of Mary Magdalene*, how back in this first century era, demons were seen as symptoms of emotional or physical illness.

This means that Mary Magdalene's miraculous healing from having these demons cast out could have been seen as a testament to her having done deep inner emotional and psychological work.

In shamanic energy medicine, these "demons" are seen as heavy energies that can take on various metaphoric forms in the World of Spirit—and these "metaphors" consists of a wounded energy and fear-based thought patterns. When we release these, through our shamanic journeying, we also release the hold this heavy energy has had on us, allowing us to heal.

But from the day when Pope Gregory announced his sudden declaration, Mary Magdalene would become known as the sinner, and repentant whore.

The Catholic Church finally admitted in 1969 that it had mistakenly identified Mary Magdalene as a prostitute, and in 2016 Pope Francis referred to her as the apostle of the apostles—as she was the one to tell the disciples the good news of Yeshua's resurrection.

Her ancient wisdom teachings rise again

As the orthodox view took over in the Christian world, other early gospels seem to have disappeared, as if they were hidden, perhaps in an effort to preserve their teachings until the time was right for them to reappear again. Some of these early gospels were discovered in 1945 when early texts dating to the first and second century were found in Nag Hammadi in Egypt. These texts include the *Gospel of Thomas* and the *Gospel of Phillip*.

The *Gospel of Mary* was also discovered in 1896, and this gospel is dated to around the same time period as the ones found in Nag Hammadi.

From these early texts, a very different picture of Mary Magdalene appears. She is described as Yeshua's companion, and the one who is most understanding of his message.

This view of her went against the patriarchal version of Christianity, so she had to be cast as sinful, her importance suppressed, and her voice silenced—just as it was with the Norse goddess Hel, who was made into the evil and scary ruler of Hell by Christianity, effectively stopping the people from worshipping her as a powerful Mother Goddess. Likewise, how the Norse goddess Freya, who was deeply loved by her people, was seen as promiscuous, wicked, and bad by Christianity, and made into the Queen of Witches while the women following her risked being sentenced for witchcraft.

But we are now awakening, reclaiming our feminine power, and we are starting to remember and recognize that Mary Magdalene was a great teacher and mystic, the one who supported Yeshua through that portal of death and rebirth. Just as the Divine Mothers do, as they are portals of life, death, and rebirth.

Yeshua gave his secret teachings to Mary Magdalene, so that she could go out there and spread the good news—the miracle of resurrection and rebirth.

Just like Mary Magdalene, you are meant to go out into the world, sharing the good news that the Wise Woman within us is awakening, guiding us to eat her fruit of wisdom, so that we can remember the truth of who we are. That we are good, that we are loving, and that we are portals of life itself.

Mary Magdalene Is the Mystical Heart Embodying Both Heaven and Earth

• • • • • •

Your heart took you on a journey through the four chambers where you met both the Dark Mothers and the Light Mothers. Mary Magdalene embodies both. She knows the depth of our grief and suffering, so she knows how to descend into the sacred darkness of the lower world, and in this way, she connects us with the Dark Mothers, through our womb chakra, helping us to witness what we are meant to heal and transform, so that we can birth something new into being.

Mary Magdalene also knows how to ascend to the magical light-filled upper world and, in this way, she connects us with the Light Mothers, through our third eye, helping us witness who we are becoming, so that we can blossom into an expanded expression of our soul's truth.

She connects us with the middle world, with our life here now, through our heart chakra, which is the portal that connects heaven and earth, the human and the divine, the darkness and the light.

And just as she trusted her mystical visions, she can help us trust what we see through the eye of our heart.

In the shamanic journey we will soon do, Mary Magdalene will guide you through a sacred initiation, where you start to see through the eye of the heart, so you can trust your inner guidance as you start to weave a new story into being—the story where you are sharing your heart's loving wisdom into your world.

The Heart Chakra of the World

· · · · · ·

In the shamanic journey with Mary Magdalene, I will guide you to the heart chakra of the world, which is in Glastonbury, England, UK, a place where I have had many spiritual awakenings. I always take my shamanic energy medicine students there as part of their training with me, so that they can experience the powerful energies found in this magical place—and you, too, will experience them in the shamanic journey.

The Isle of Avalon

According to legend, Glastonbury is the Isle of Avalon, which is not so strange, as two thousand years ago, the surrounding land was marshland, and parts of Glastonbury would have been an actual island.

This is the mythical land of King Arthur, Guinevere and Merlin, and Glastonbury has long been seen as the gateway to the Celtic Otherworld.

Britain's first monastery was built here in A.D. 63, and many believe that Joseph of Arimathea brought Mary Magdalene and Mother Mary to Glastonbury after Yeshua's death.

The ley lines of Mary and Archangel Michael cross near the High Altar in Glastonbury Abbey, and this crossing represents the sacred marriage of the divine feminine and the divine masculine.

You also find two sacred wells here—the Red Spring and the White Spring. In the Red Spring flows the holy water of the divine feminine, and this spring feeds the sacred well in the beautiful Chalice Well Gardens. In the White Spring flows the holy water of the divine masculine.

These two springs nearly join, at the foot of the Tor, a sacred hill in Glastonbury, which is believed to be the original Isle of Avalon. On the side of this beautiful hill grow apple trees and Avalon is the Isle of Apples. As we know, apples can be seen as the fruit of feminine wisdom and magic.

The Tor used to be a centre for rites and initiations of druid priests and priestesses, and people have been making pilgrimages to this holy place for over one thousand years.

Glastonbury is a very magical place, and in this shamanic journey, you'll be taken there, connecting you with the Red Spring (divine feminine), the Tor (a hill that is the gateway to the Otherworld), and the White Spring (divine masculine).

Shamanic Journey with Mary Magdalene to the Heart Chakra of the World—the Isle of Avalon

• • • • • •

Let us do a shamanic journey now, where your journey guide will be Mary Magdalene, as she is the mystical heart embodying both heaven and earth.

In this way, she can help you to dance with the seasons of darkness and light, seeing through the eye of your heart, while weaving your heart's loving wisdom into your life.

On this journey you will be guided to the Isle of Avalon, the heart chakra of the world, so that you can experience the powerful energies found in this magical place.

I strongly recommend that you let me guide you through this journey by listening to my voice guiding you through it. You can access the recording of this journey on **cissiwilliams.com/heart**. It is 34 minutes long.

Shamanic Journey with Mary Magdalene to the Heart Chakra of the World—the Isle of Avalon

Close your eyes and sink into your inner stillness.

Sink deeper into your mystical heart, where you see a beautiful light shining. A light that is a portal into the World of Spirit.

Journey through the portal into the World of Spirit

Take a deep breath in. As you breathe out, feel how you journey through this portal now, into the World of Spirit, where you find yourself in an ancient forest.

You notice there is a path in front of you, a path that is leading through the forest and, as you start walking on this path, you can hear the gentle sound of birds singing, as if they are welcoming you to this sacred place.

You keep walking, deeper and deeper into the forest, until you come to a cave—a cave that is a doorway into the divine feminine.

Meeting Mary Magdalene

By the entrance to this cave, you meet Mary Magdalene. She is beautiful, and her heart chakra is radiant, like a holy flame glowing from the essence of eternal love, ancient wisdom, and fierce compassion.

Mary Magdalene takes your hand and leads you through the entrance of this cave, into a dark chamber, with a spiralling staircase leading down.

You start walking down this staircase, spiralling down into the core of the earth, deeper and deeper into the heart of the Great Mother, until you reach an underground river, a river of light. There is a beautiful mist dancing over the river, a mist that is the mystical presence of the goddess.

Journey to the Isle of Avalon

There is a boat here, and as you step inside this boat, it starts to carry you on this river of light, through the mist—deeper and deeper into the sacred landscape of the feminine.

After a while the river leads you out into the ocean, where the mist parts, allowing you to see a green island in the distance.

This is the Isle of Avalon, the sacred island that is the gateway to the Otherworld. The boat carries you all the way to the island and, as you arrive, you step out of the boat.

You start walking on a tiny path that is leading you into the centre of the island, to a hill that rises majestically towards the heavens.

As you reach the hill, the path starts to circle upwards, and you keep following the path, spiralling up the hill, until you reach a gateway—like a shimmering veil.

Entering the ancient apple orchard of the goddess

Take a deep breath in and, as you breathe out, pierce through this veil, and step through the gateway and into an ancient apple orchard.

This orchard is a sacred paradise of the goddess, filled with feminine magic, divine wisdom, and healing medicine. You see hundreds of lush apple trees, all bearing the fruits of the goddess.

There is a circle of women here in the orchard—a circle filled with all your sisters, Wise Women, and ancient wise witches that you have met on your journey—both from this world and from the Otherworld.

They are all here, welcoming you to this magical place.

But before you can enter their sacred circle, you first have to step through a portal of fire, a mystical gateway you need to pass through, before you can be initiated into the wisdom of the goddess.

Releasing the fears

Mary Magdalene asks you to witness all the fears you carry within you; fears of being seen, fears of speaking your truth, and fears of showing up in the world as the Wise Woman that you are.

Notice these fears now, and then step into this portal of fire. Feel how the holy fire burns these old fears away, transforming them into light, releasing you from that old hold.

Step through this portal now, through this mystical gateway, into a new expansion of your feminine power, magic, and wisdom.

As you emerge through the portal you can hear all your sisters, all the Wise Women and ancient witches singing, celebrating your return to their sacred circle.

Mary Magdalene now leads you to a well that is filled with the holy waters of the divine feminine. It is as if the water is sparkling from the light-filled essence of the creative feminine magic—the light-filled essence that births life itself.

Receiving medicine from the four elements

As you lie down in this well, feel how the light-filled waters start to heal you, cleanse you, and rejuvenate you.

These holy waters connect you with the sacred rivers and wells of the Divine Mother, helping you to always move with the flow of life, whilst being supported and guided by her.

As you are floating on these holy waters, feel the grounding energy of the earth beneath you, and trust that you are always being held in the loving arms of the Divine Mother, wherever you are in life.

Hear the wind blowing in the trees, whispering to you words of wisdom from the Ancient Mother. It is as if the wind is her breath and, as you breathe in, you are breathing in her wisdom and, as you breathe out, feel how you are expressing her wisdom through you and out into the world.

As you are floating on these sacred waters, notice how the Heavens open, allowing the golden light from the Sun to flow directly into you, igniting your higher consciousness in your third eye, so you can see through the eyes of wisdom; igniting the divine flame in your heart, so you can perceive through the eye of the heart; and igniting the magic in your womb chakra, so you can birth your dreams into being.

Feel how the light from the Moon and the stars, and from the Aurora Borealis, flows directly into you, filling you with the healing light from the sacred darkness of the night.

Let yourself be nourished by all this medicine from the Heavens and the Earth.

The cloak and the apple

Now step out of the well and, as you do, you receive a beautiful cloak from Mary Magdalene—a cloak that connects you with this ancient source of feminine magic—a magic that protects you, holds you, sustains you, and guides you.

Mary Magdalene gives you an apple from one of the holy trees growing in this orchard—an apple that is filled with the wisdom of the goddess.

As you bite into this apple, let it reveal to you the feminine wisdom you are meant to embody.

As this wisdom is revealed to you, you can hear all your sisters, all the Wise Women and ancient witches celebrating you, as you remember this feminine wisdom you are meant to be an expression of.

Awakening the eye in your heart

Mary Magdalene now touches your heart, awakening the eye in your heart and, as it awakens, your heart starts to glow from a beautiful divine light, like a holy flame filled with love and fierce compassion.

Mary Magdalene asks you to notice how in the past, humanity has been stuck in a false perception of the feminine, looking through the eyes of fear and judgment—and, as you now have awakened the eye in your heart, she wants you to witness the ancient feminine wisdom through the eye of the heart.

Notice what you see, as you look through the eye of the heart at all the women gathered here—all your sisters, Wise Women, and ancient witches.

See their light, see their magic, see their love, see their feminine power.

Now see yourself, through the eye of the heart. Allow yourself to witness your light, your magic, your love, your feminine power.

Journey to the Red and White Spring

Mary Magdalene now takes your hand and together you start walking out of the apple orchard, onto a little path that is leading through a beautiful forest, filled with wildflowers, berries and ancient trees, until you come to a rose garden.

Here in this rose garden flows the Red Spring, the holy waters of the Divine Feminine. Hear the gentle bubbling sound from the White Spring, the holy waters of the Divine Masculine.

Becoming the Tree of Life

Mary Magdalene walks with you to the heart of the well of the Divine Feminine. As you stand here by this holy well, a place that's been visited for thousands of years by those who have heard her call – the call of the Divine Mother—feel how you become like a Tree of Life, with your roots going deep down into the earth, connecting you with your ancestors, with the magic and wisdom held in the sacred darkness, with the Dark Mothers and their healing medicine for you.

Feel how your roots on the left search for the holy waters of the Red Spring, the flowing waters of the healthy divine feminine. Let your roots on the left absorb all the medicine that is here for you, from the healthy divine feminine.

Feel how your roots on the right search for the holy waters of the White Spring, the flowing waters of the healthy divine masculine. Let your roots on the right absorb all the medicine that is here for you, from the healthy divine masculine.

Now tune into your branches, and feel how they reach high up into the sky, connecting you with that which you are becoming, with the sun and the moon and the stars, with the magical light of the heavens, with the Light Mothers, and their healing medicine for you.

Your Tree of Life helps you to tune into the different domains of reality—you tune into the lower world through the roots; into the upper world through the branches; and into the middle world through the trunk of the tree.

Weaving magic and wisdom from your womb chakra

Now tune into your womb chakra and feel how you start to weave your love, feminine wisdom, and magic into the lower world—into the unconscious mind of your loved ones, into the mythical landscape of your soul and of the feminine—the landscape where we are all held in the loving arms of the Dark Mother.

Weave all your healing medicine from your womb chakra to all your loved ones, filling your relationships with a golden healing light—so it flows into the depth of your relationships, to the root of your love, to a connection that is so deep you can't see it with your physical eyes, but you can feel this connection in your soul.

Now weave in all your love and wisdom and feminine magic into your important life areas—into the depth of all these areas, filling them with this golden healing light, at this deeper soul level.

Weaving magic and wisdom from your third eye

Now tune into your third eye and feel how you start to weave your love, feminine wisdom, and magic into the upper world—into the higher consciousness of your loved ones, into the mythical landscape of Spirit, of that which you are becoming—the landscape where we are all held in the loving arms of the Light Mother.

Weave all your healing medicine from your third eye into your connection with all your loved ones, into the highest divine potential of your relationships, the highest expression of your love. An expression that is so much more than what your mind could ever know—but Spirit knows what this highest expression is.

Weave in all your love and wisdom and feminine magic into your important life areas—to the highest expression of love within all these areas, filling them with all this light, allowing them to blossom into their highest divine potential.

Weaving magic and wisdom from your heart chakra

Now tune into your heart chakra, to the eye of your heart, and feel how you start to weave your love, wisdom, and feminine magic into the middle world, so into the mythical landscape of your life—the landscape where we are all held in the loving arms of Mother Earth, as she dances with the seasons of darkness and light.

Weave all your healing medicine from the eye of your heart to all your loved ones—filling your relationships with a golden, healing light—into the heart of your relationships, into the love that is always there, like a divine flame burning so brightly.

Now weave all your love, wisdom, and feminine magic into the important areas of your life—to the heart of all these areas, filling them with a golden light from your heart.

Your fruits of feminine wisdom and magic

Notice, how your Tree of Life—that is rooted deep into the earth of this rose garden in the heart chakra of the world—is filled with beautiful fruits that are glowing from a golden light; a light that is the essence of feminine wisdom and magic.

Mary Magdalene explains that these are the fruits you are meant to share with others, fruits that have developed through your own deep healing and awakening of this ancient, loving, magical feminine power that lives within you.

She gives you a basket and instructs you to fill it with all these light-filled fruits that you are meant to share with others.

Then say goodbye to Mary Magdalene and let us prepare to journey back.

Journey back through the portal

Take a deep breath in and, as you breathe out, feel how you journey into the portal that is leading into your mystical heart.

Take another deep breath in and, as you breathe out, feel how you journey through this portal now, bringing your fruits of wisdom, and all your gifts with you, into your body, into the here and now.

Take another deep breath in and, as you breathe out, feel how you now journey into your life, sharing your light-filled fruits of wisdom and feminine magic with those you love.

Take another deep breath in and, as you breathe out, you can open your eyes.

◡

Take a few moments now to write down all your insights and learnings, gifts, and messages.

If you want to, write a letter to yourself, from your heart, and perhaps also from Mary Magdalene, so that they can share with you their messages and advice. By doing this you are re-writing your own story, filling your new life story with wisdom teachings, feminine power, and magic, where you are sharing your soul gifts, fruits of wisdom and healing medicine with others.

You can start the letter with the words:

What my heart and Mary Magdalene want me to know is …

Then put the book down and give yourself some sacred time to reflect upon all the healing you have just experienced.

Living a Heart-Centred Life

Let your heart guide you ... it whispers, so listen closely.
— WALT DISNEY

I t is now time to bring your heart's dreams into your physical reality, so that you can live a heart-centred life, instead of letting them stay stuck as lofty ideas in your thoughts.

And to do this, you must learn how to harness the power of your time, energy, and focus, because when you lack this ability, you won't be able to give your heart's dreams the nourishment they need to manifest in your life.

I learnt this very important lesson from my dad.

A container filled with dreams

My dad was a dreamer, and one of his dreams was to build us a bigger house, so that we could all live with him. He loved freedom and the outdoors, so he never lived in our flat. Instead, he spent his time in our tiny wooden summer house, which had no running water, bathroom facilities, or proper heating (only a fireplace).

Although the house lacked modern luxuries, the land it was situated on was beautiful, with its own woodland of birch and pine trees, blueberry bushes, wildflowers, and soft moss covering the ground.

Dad had this dream of us all living together in a house with a downstairs and an upstairs. He started the building work and created a whole new foundation, which had a basement for the downstairs bathroom and bedrooms. He even moved our old house, so it was on top of this new basement. He drilled for water and installed a water tank, so we had access to running water. But then his energy fizzled out. The bathroom was never installed, and the basement remained unfinished.

When he died (in 2004) we found unopened boxes of the most expensive tiles, wallpaper, and bathroom suite my dad could afford—all from the seventies. All his dreams were stored away in this container, as he had been unable to use his time, energy, and focus effectively. Instead, the vodka demon would get him, often by lunchtime. He ended up living in an unfinished house, alone. And every time, as he looked out through the window, he would see this container—a reminder of what could have been.

I am a dreamer, just like my dad. Fortunately, I was blessed to have him in my life, so I could see first-hand what happens when we waste our time, energy, and focus as well as seeing the consequences of us not healing our inner wounds. I learnt to become very discerning in what I give my time and energy to, and what I choose to focus upon, and I will soon share how you can do that too.

This will help you find the *structure* you need to birth your dreams into the world. If you don't have a good structure, then nothing can be born—just as an embryo needs the structure and support of the womb around it to develop into a baby, you need the structure of a strong inner cauldron for your dreams to fully form, as this cauldron is the container of your feminine magic, power, and creativity. If the cauldron is leaking, then you are leaking life force, making it hard for your dreams to get the nourishment they need.

This means that if we don't show up in creating the *structure* that can birth our dreams into the world, they will never materialize. They will just stay as lofty ideas in the ether—or stuck in a container filled with unrealized dreams. And that is so frustrating, because we can feel we are meant to be the conduit that brings them through from the Divine Source, into our physical reality.

I will soon give you three inquiry questions you can use to focus your time and energy in such a way that you turn your heart's loving dreams into reality. And to help you with this, we will call in the powerful

Valkyries—Norse female warriors that are bringers of light. They know a thing or two about how to focus your time and energy so that you can show up for the action needed in your life.

Flying with the Valkyries

Thanks to my dad showing me what happens when we don't use our time, energy, and focus wisely, I've become ultra-committed to making the most of the time and energy I have. What has really helped me is to call in the Valkyries—powerful female warriors bringers of light.

The Valkyries

Freya is actually the head Valkyrie—some see her as the Queen of the Valkyries—as she gets the first pick of the fallen soldiers and takes them to Folkvangr, her heavenly field. Then she sends the other half to Odin, in Valhalla.

This is the aspect of Freya, called Valfreya, who helps us to make wiser choices—the word *val* in Swedish means *choice*.

The Valkyries from the Norse sagas radiate light as they ride through the sky, brightening up the world. They have solar goddess qualities. They are the embodiment of powerful feminine energy, showing us how to fly over the battlefields, noticing which battles to let go of and which ones to engage in. In this way they help us use our *discernment* so that we can *choose wisely*.

The Valkyries know we often get stuck in battles—dramas, conflicts, problems—that we are just not meant to get sucked into, as it will drain us of energy. Just as a warrior can't fight every battle, we too must learn which ones to pick. However, once we are called to engage in a battle—a difficult situation—then we must engage fully. There is no such thing as a half-hearted battle.

The Valkyries have taught me that when I'm faced with a problem I'm meant to engage in, I need to do so with a hundred percent of my energy and focus. This often solves the problem quickly, as I'm fully committed.

The Valkyries are no light and fluffy light bringers; they are female warriors, so they can show you, in a "kick-some-ass" sort of way, how to release from your life activities, situations, and relationships that are not in alignment with your highest path. This releases you from what has previously drained you, so that you can instead invest your time, energy, and focus into what helps to light up your world.

Flying over the battlefield

The Valkyries fly over the battlefield, picking up the fallen soldiers, taking them into the afterlife.

This means that these female warriors help us move through the portal of death into rebirth, assisting us in letting go of that which is no longer working, so that we have more time, energy, and focus available for what we are meant to birth in our lives.

Whenever you notice you are stuck, and you know this aspect of your life is meant to be released, hand it over to the Valkyries so they can assist you in moving through that portal.

The norn of the future, Skuld, is actually a Valkyrie, so she helps us weave something new into being—that which "shall be." But for that future to become realized, we first must be willing to move through the portal of death and rebirth.

INQUIRY: Questions with the Valkyries

The Valkyries can help you become more aware of your energetic leaks and how you are meant to focus your time and energy, by you noticing the following (write down your answers):

- Which battles are you meant to let go of—situations, activities, relationships—that you know in your heart are not in alignment with your highest path?

- How are you wasting your time, energy, and focus?

- How can you focus your time and energy more wisely?

Look at what you've written and notice what stands out. Whatever energetic leaks you've discovered, take steps to amend them—and hand them over to the Valkyries in the shamanic journey at the end of this chapter.

Make sure to create space for activities you know are in alignment with how you are meant to invest your time, energy, and focus.

By doing this, you allow your dreams to receive the nourishment and structure they need so they can become materialized.

Listening to the Whispers from Your Heart

After having discovered how you can use your time, energy, and focus with more wisdom, the next step is to look at how to receive guidance on what action is needed to turn your dreams into reality.

They key here is to make sure that the guidance is from your heart and not from the ego-mind.

Your heart knows how to guide you to the blossoming and expansion of all that you are meant to be, as your heart is in sync with your soul's vision for your life.

As you tune into your heart, it will show you how you can lovingly embrace the changes of the seasons. It will guide you to let go in the autumn and retreat into the darkness of winter, to then open up to receive the magical light of spring, so you can blossom into your next greatest expression of life in the summer.

Your heart knows how to assist you in the unfolding of your highest path, as it beats in rhythm to the heartbeat of the Great Mother, singing the ancient song of the Wise Woman, so you can awaken her wild feminine wisdom within you.

Your heart is the container that holds your ancestors' wisdom from the past and your soul's vision of the future—and the Wise Woman, who flows through your veins, is the Spirit Weaver who has come forth into this time–space reality to help weave your dreams into being.

Your heart knows how to guide you to birth those dreams that are for the highest good of all, while the ego-mind hasn't got a clue, as it is only interested in "what's in it for me."

Unfortunately, when we start learning about goalsetting, it is usually all from the ego-mind. Let me explain what I mean.

A healed mind does not plan

Having seen how my dad wasted his time, energy, and focus, I became very good at setting goals and creating an action plan. Hence, it made me really frustrated when I kept opening the same page in *A Course in Miracles* where I read:

> *A healed mind does not plan. It carries out the plans that it receives through listening to wisdom that is not its own. It waits until it has been taught what should be done and then proceeds to do it.*

When I read this the first time, I was like, "What do you mean I am not meant to plan?"

It just did not make sense to me, especially since I had seen what happened with my dad, who did not stick to a plan. But as I kept on reading, I realized that what *A Course in Miracles* meant was that *any self-initiated plans are from the ego-mind.*

This is because the ego-mind keeps regurgitating the same old, same old, from the past and into the future, which keeps us trapped in time, so any goals from the ego-mind would just repeat what I already knew.

If I wanted to create something *new*, if I wanted to weave my heart's dreams into being and allow my soul's vision for my life to unfold, then I needed to be willing to listen to a wiser voice—the voice of the Divine Intelligence flowing through my veins, wired into my DNA, and embedded within my bones. To listen to the voice of the Wise Woman within, who speaks to me through the whispers of my heart.

By tuning into HER guidance, I started to take inspired action that led me to where I am today. My life is totally different, compared to how it was before I listened to her voice. In the past, I tried to manifest from my head, constantly chasing the light. And I was quite good at it, but it was exhausting.

These days, I listen to the whispers of my heart, tuning into the guidance from the Wise Woman within. I let her lead me, guiding me on where to go, what to do, what to say, and to whom. I dance with the sacred darkness and the magical light, and it has allowed my life to unfold and blossom in the most miraculous way.

And it will do this for you too. As you listen to her voice guiding you, as you embrace the medicine of the darkness and the light, then the future that unfolds will be so much better than what the ego-mind could ever dream of. And that's how you create a future unlike the past. That's how you unhook yourself from the ego-mind's need to control, by being willing to be guided by this ancient, wise, loving presence that knows how to lead you to your highest path—a path that unfolds in an organic and magical way, for the highest good of all.

The Wise Woman within you is the ancient "witch-within-wood," the primordial darkness that births the light, and the magical light that nourishes all of life. She is the Loving Presence that guides the seasons, helping you to let go of the old so that you can invite the new. She is you and you are her, as she is life itself.

The ego-mind is not you—it holds a belief that you are separate from life—while the Wise Woman within you knows you are intricately connected with all of creation.

All of the exercises and shamanic journeys in this book have helped you to remove what has blocked you from listening to this wise, loving inner voice. And you know you are listening to her when you feel peaceful, loving, compassionate, and connected with others. You know you are listening to the voice of the ego when you feel agitated, righteous, judgmental, and separate from others.

And this difference was huge for me to understand when it came to *planning and taking action*. Yes, I was good at planning and taking action, as I had seen from my dad what happens when you don't. But the way I was planning and taking action was still from fear, so it was still from the ego-mind, focusing on the past. I didn't want to be like my dad, so I kept chasing the light, I kept chasing the dreams of the future by frantically taking action.

As I shifted my focus, I stopped listening to my mind that was constantly looking at the future; I stopped chasing.

Instead, I tuned into my heart's loving wisdom.

I released what I was meant to let go of, including my mind's addiction to constantly focusing on the future.

I stopped planning.

Instead, I allowed myself to journey into the sacred darkness, resting in the Dark Mother's loving arms. I gave myself time to pause.

I waited. And waited. And waited.

Until the guidance suddenly came through. I felt this guidance as an inner knowing, like a gentle nudge—*read this book, contact this person, do this course, take this action.* As I followed the guidance, a new path opened up. The path where I was listening to the whispers of my heart guiding me toward living a heart-led life.

If I hadn't shifted my focus from my mind to my heart, from the outer to the inner, from constantly chasing the light—with my mind—to instead journeying into the sacred darkness waiting to *receive* the light— in the form of guidance, dreams, visions, soul gifts, healing medicine—I would never have started to teach shamanic energy medicine, founded the podcast, or written this book.

As long as I kept chasing the light, I was trapped in the Western mind's addiction of always having to be in a perpetual spring and summer, where we are planting new ideas, achieving, manifesting, and harvesting. But life doesn't grow like that. A seed can only grow into a tree by first being planted in the darkness of moist soil. It grows roots down into the earth to receive nourishment.

At the same time, it grows upwards as a green shoot to receive the light from the life-giving rays of the sun. By embracing the medicine from both the darkness and the light, it can grow into a plant.

The tree also needs a period of stillness in the autumn and winter, when it's resting in the Dark Mother's loving arms, receiving the nourishment it needs, as it waits for the light to return. It is this resting that allows it to grow for each season.

It is the same with us—we grow as we allow ourselves to rest, which is reflected in how the body heals and grows in our sleep.

When we keep chasing the light, we never rest in the stillness of the sacred darkness. And it is only in this stillness that we can hear the whispers from our loving heart.

Your heart knows what is best for you, as your heart looks after *you*. And your heart wants you to be all that you are meant to be, in a way that is sustainable for you.

Trust that when you pause to listen to your heart's loving voice, the guidance will come. And once the guidance comes, and you start to take heart-inspired action, you will be guided to the path where you shine your light and share your soul gifts, dreams, and healing medicine with others. And your heart is the compass that always guides you to the highest unfolding of this path.

Tuning into the whispers of your heart

How can you then tune into the whispers of your heart?

Anytime you allow yourself to be in the present moment, you tune into your heart.

Perhaps you find that you are completely present in the now when you are doing yoga, meditating, playing a musical instrument, walking in nature, sitting on a beach listening to the waves crashing into the shore, holding a baby, stroking a pet, writing in a journal, or any other activity that takes you out of the mind's focus on the past or the future, so that you can instead just be, present, in the here and now. All of this helps you to tune into your heart.

And when you want to set aside a few minutes to consciously connect with your heart's loving wisdom, you can do the following exercise.

◼ **EXERCISE to Tune Into Your Heart's Whispers**

- Set aside time when you can be undisturbed, so you allow yourself the sacred space you need to retreat into the silence within your mystical heart.

- Sit in a comfortable position, with a pen and a journal in your lap.

- Close your eyes, place a hand on your heart.

- Take a deep breath in and, as you breathe out, feel how you sink into the stillness within your mystical heart.

- Take another deep breath in, and as you breathe out, tune into the light that shines in your mystical heart. This light is the loving wisdom of your heart.

- Then open your eyes, and now pick up your pen and journal. Tune within and say to yourself:

What my heart wants me to know is ...

Then write down the answers. Keep writing for as long as you feel the loving energy from your heart flowing through you. Your heart may give you advice on various areas of your life—your relationships, your health, your business. Trust it. Your heart is very wise, and it loves you. It is connected with all of life, so it will only guide you to that which is for the highest good of all.

By regularly tuning into the loving wisdom in your heart, you start to tune into the Wise Woman within, so that she can guide you, with every heartbeat, to dance with the full spectrum of life—the darkness and the light.

She'll whisper to you when it's time to retreat inward, letting go of that which you no longer need. She'll hold you in a loving embrace as you rest in the sacred darkness, waiting for the light to return. And as the first seeds, the light of new dreams, appear, she'll encourage you to receive them, so you can become pregnant with this new life. She'll also guide you as to how you can best nourish these divine dreams within you, so that they can grow. And then, she'll be the midwife, helping you to birth them into the world, so that they can be shared with others.

She knows every stage of this magical cycle of creation is sacred, as all of it is following the beautiful drumbeat of the everchanging seasons of the sacred darkness and magical light.

As you now have started to tune into the loving wisdom of your heart, it is time to look at the steps you need to take, as you listen to its guidance. In this way, you discover the structure you need to birth your dreams and soul gifts into the world.

Finding the Structure for Birthing Your Dreams

Your heart knows how to guide you to the path you are meant to take, as your heart is always in tune with life all around you, with the seasons and the elements, and with the Wise Woman within.

Let this Wise Woman now step forth, by answering the following questions, so that you can receive from her the structure you need for your dreams to be born.

EXERCISE for Finding the Structure for Birthing Your Dreams

- Set aside time when you can be undisturbed, so you allow yourself the sacred space you need to retreat into the silence within your mystical heart.

- Sit in a comfortable position, with a pen and a journal in your lap.

- Close your eyes, and tune into your heart.

- Take a deep breath in and, as you breathe out, feel how you sink into the light that shines within your mystical heart.

- Take another deep breath in and, as you breathe out, feel how you sink even deeper into the light, into the presence of love that lives in your heart—the Wise Woman within you. This is the one who dances with the seasons of darkness and light.

- Take another deep breath in and, as you do that, feel how you connect with her, and how *she breathes into you*, syncing your breath together so that as you breathe out, you are both breathing together.

- Her breath is your breath. Your breath is her breath.

From this place, open your eyes, pick up your pen and journal, and let the Wise Woman within you answer the following questions—write down her answers to you:

- What are the soul gifts, healing medicine, and dreams you want me to share with the world?

- How can I create space for this to grow?

- Which is the soul gift, dream, or healing medicine I'm meant to focus on the most, in the next coming few months?

- How do I need to structure my time, so I make sure I have the energy needed to birth this into the world?

- What do I need to focus on?

- Which action do I need to take this week, this month, in the next three months, and in this coming year, to create a structure that supports me in weaving this into my life and my world?

- What is the very first step I need to begin with?

- As you write down these answers, you start to discover the *structure* needed for this to manifest, so you move it from being a thought, into reality.

227

Trust that as you act on that very first step, and then the next one, and the next one, you start to weave the loving wisdom from the Wise Woman within you into your life. She is the midwife that helps to birth your soul gifts, dreams, and healing medicine into your world.

Now tune into your inner wisdom, place one hand over your heart, and ask yourself the following question:

What is my new commitment to my heart that will help
me with all of this?

Write this new commitment down. As you act on this new commitment by taking the structured, inspired action needed to weave all these light-filled dreams and powerful healing medicine into the world, you weave your heart's loving wisdom into your life.

But it all starts with taking that one first step, while listening to the whispers from your heart, and following the guidance from the Wise Woman within. And then the next step. And then the next step.

Let us now do our final shamanic journey in which you start to weave all this magic, wisdom, and healing medicine into your world.

Shamanic Journey to Weave Your Heart's Loving Wisdom into Your World

Let us take our final shamanic journey, where you'll again journey to the Tree of Life. Here you'll tune into how your roots connect with the underworld and the Dark Mothers, helping you to heal your past; your branches connect you with the upper world, with the Light Mothers, with new dreams and visions; and your heart chakra connects you with the middle world, as it acts as the portal between heaven and earth, so that you can bring all this wisdom and light out into your life.

You may remember that within the trunk of the tree lies the ancient feminine wisdom the Norse Sagas called "the witch-within-wood." She is the one who has now been awakened within you. She is the healer, the seer, the *völva*, the witch, the spiritual midwife, who knows how to assist you in birthing and weaving a new consciousness into your world.

She is the Wise Woman within, and you connect with her both through your bones—as in the Tree of Life—*and* through the seasons of darkness and light that flow in sync with your heartbeat.

There is a natural relationship between the bones and the heart, as new blood is being formed in the bone marrow of the long bones of the body, just as there is a natural connection between the Tree of Life and your heart through the seasons. Plus, the heart chakra links the lower world and the upper world, so it is the portal that connects you with your roots and your ancestors, and with the branches that expand into the light of who you are becoming.

The Wise Woman lives within your bones and in your heart. She's the witch-within-wood, the primordial mother who guides the seasons of darkness and light, and she is the Ancient Mother that sustains you from within, through your blood.

She is living within you, in your DNA. She is you, and you are her, and it is now time for the Wise Woman that you are to step forth, and weave your magic, soul gifts, and healing medicine into your world.

On this journey, you will meet the norns again, and you'll meet the Valkyries. You will also meet the Norse goddess Saga. Her name means "the one who sees," as she can see into the future by tracking the strands of what is coming.

In Swedish *saga* means "story." Thus, she is a goddess who can help us let go of the old stories, so that we can instead weave and spin new stories for the future, by becoming conscious of the energy we use with our words, thoughts, and actions.

Saga lives by a little river, Sökkvabäck, and Odin used to like visiting her, where she would offer him a drink from her golden cup.

Jacob Grimm, who together with his brother wrote down many of the ancient European folk tales, felt this was a drink of immortality and poetry. In this way, it is similar to the Celtic drink of Awen, as well as to the essence of the golden apples from Idun.

In this journey, Saga will help you to create a new story for the future—a story of the Wise Woman, a story where you are weaving your heart's loving wisdom into your world.

I strongly recommend that you listen to my voice guiding you through this shamanic journey. You can access it on **cissiwilliams.com/heart**. It is 38 minutes long.

Shamanic Journey to Weave Your Heart's Loving Wisdom into Your World

Sit or lie down in a comfortable position. Close your eyes and sink into your inner stillness.

Sink deeper and deeper into the stillness in your mystical heart, where there is a light shining. This light is a portal that leads into the World of Spirit.

Journey through the portal

Take a deep breath in and, as you breathe out, feel how you journey through this portal into the World of Spirit, where you find yourself in an ancient forest.

Here, in this forest, you notice how you are becoming like a tree—the Tree of Life—and your tree is in full bloom. All around you, the forest is buzzing with life. The sun's golden light is streaming through the treetops, the birds are singing, and the air is filled with the refreshing scent of birch trees, pine needles, and wildflowers.

Tune into your roots

Your tree is beautiful and strong, with the roots going deep down into the sacred darkness, deep into the earth. Feel how your roots are drawing up a healing, energizing, loving energy from the Dark Mother, filling you with her love, her support, and her sustenance for you. Let this lifegiving energy flow up your roots and into you—into your bones.

Tune into your bone marrow within your bones and feel how new blood is being formed here—healthy, loving, supportive, nourishing blood from the Dark Mother. Feel how this new loving blood flows into your whole body, filling you with her love *from within your bones*.

Let your roots go even deeper into the earth, so deep that they connect you with your ancestors, and with your other sisters who are also awakening this ancient wisdom within them. Feel how there is a collective of roots of awakening, of remembering, like a collective web of wisdom, magic, and ancient feminine power, here in the sacred darkness of the earth.

The Dark Mother now shares with you her wisdom and advice for you—so let yourself receive all this wisdom from her now.

Tune into your branches

Tune into the branches of your tree. Notice how they stretch far up into the sky, opening up to receive the light from above, from the upper world, from the Divine Source of all that is.

Feel how your branches connect you with that which you are becoming, with the sun and the moon and the stars, with the magical light of the heavens, with the Light Mothers and their healing medicine for you.

Let yourself receive all of this light now—through the branches of your tree. Let this light of new healing, insights, visions, and dreams flow into your branches, and into your consciousness.

Let yourself receive the light of new beginnings, hope, and healing medicine from the Light Mothers.

Keep breathing all this light in, breathing in this expansion of life. Let it fill you up. Let this light flow in through the branches and into the trunk of the tree.

The Light Mothers now share with you their wisdom and advice for you—so let yourself receive all this wisdom now.

The Tree of Life as a staff

Your Tree of Life is the connection with the World of Spirit. It is like a staff that helps you to travel into the different worlds of reality— into the lower world through the roots; into the upper world through the branches; and into the middle world through the trunk of the tree.

The Wise Woman within the tree

Feel how you are inside this tree as if you are the Wise Woman within the tree—the ancient witch-within-wood that existed before time. Feel, see, and experience how this ancient witch, this Wise Woman within, opens her eyes.

She now starts to breathe her wisdom, magic, and power into you, awakening you. "Remember," she says, "remember who you are."

And you remember. You can feel this power, magic, and wisdom rise, rise, rise within you.

You can feel the medicine of the sacred darkness flow up your roots and into you, and the medicine from the magical light from the heavens flow into you—and you remember.

You remember you are the conduit of darkness and light, the one that births life itself. You remember that you are ancient, that you existed before time itself.

You remember that you are here to be the light in the darkness, to help share your healing medicine with the world.

You are the Wise Woman, and you are awake.

Step out of the tree as the Wise Woman

As the Wise Woman, you now step out of the tree, holding a staff in your hand—a staff that represents the Tree of Life.

Let this staff touch the earth, so it becomes filled with the healing medicine from the Earth, from your ancestors, from the Dark Mothers, filling it with power, wisdom, transformation, and magic, and with all the healing medicine of the sacred darkness.

Let this staff also become filled with the light from the heavens, from the sun and the moon and the stars, from the Divine Source, from the Light Mothers, filling your staff with the light of a new consciousness, with the power to light up our world.

Now breathe into this staff all the medicine you've received during this journey of healing, transformation, magic, and rebirth—all the learnings and insights, all the visions and dreams, all the wisdom you've received from the World of Spirit.

Know that this staff is your magical tool that helps you to journey into the World of Spirit, and it also helps you to weave light, love, wisdom, and healing medicine into the world.

As you are holding your staff, feel how you are ready and willing to serve, from this ancient medicine of being the Wise Woman.

Meeting the three norns

Notice now how the three norns, the sisters of time, are here in the ancient forest.

You have: the norn of the past, Urd; the norn of the present, Verdandi; and the norn of the future, Skuld.

Journey with Urd

The norn of the past, Urd now steps forth, spinning a thread between her fingers, a thread that leads into the past. She invites you to journey with her into the past, filling your past with all your wisdom, light, compassion, learnings, and insights, so that your past starts to shimmer and glow from a beautiful radiant light.

Journey with Urd now into the past, transforming it into a beautiful glowing light.

As your past is glowing with this radiant light, you can see your wise ancestors come up to you—thanking you for having done this journey of healing.

Urd now brings you back to the tree.

Journey with Verdandi

The norn of the present, Verdandi, now steps forth. She starts to spin a thread, inviting you to fill your present life with all your wisdom, light, soul gifts, and healing medicine.

Verdandi also shows you how you can choose to focus your time and energy better, so you allow all this wisdom, light, healing medicine, and soul gifts the energy, time, and focus they need for them to grow—so they can be brought out into the world through you.

Verdandi now brings you back to the tree.

Meeting the Valkyries

The norn of the future, Skuld, now steps forth. She is actually a Valkyrie, a light bringer, and she calls on her Valkyrie sisters. See, feel, and hear how they come flying across the sky, these beautiful light-bringers, brightening up the world wherever they go.

The Valkyries are female warriors of light—they now scoop you up, so you start flying with them, high up into the cosmos. Feel how you fly with them, on your staff—you are riding with the Valkyries—out into the future.

They show you how you can use your time, energy, and focus with more discernment, so you can be a Light Bringer—one that helps to light up the world—in a way that is in alignment with your heart's wisdom.

Feel the power of the Valkyries, their light, their commitment to being the light bringers of the world—let them ignite this light, this commitment, and this power within you. Trust that YOU are this light. You are meant to be like a shining sun, a radiant star, brightening up the world wherever you go.

The Valkyries now fly you back to the tree in the forest, where you again meet the norns.

Journey with Skuld

The norn of the future, Skuld, now starts to spin a thread where she reveals to you your highest path—the path where you are saying YES to that which lights you up, the path where you are weaving all your light, visions, dreams, and healing medicine into the world.

As you are weaving all of this into the future, also notice the next few steps you need to take—the action that is in alignment with your loving heart—so you can weave all of this into being.

Skuld now brings you back to the tree, and as you stand here by the tree you now notice that there is a path here. You start to follow this path, taking you down to a beautiful little river, with flowing waters that seem to glow from a radiant golden light.

Meeting the Norse Goddess, Saga

By this river, you meet a goddess with long golden hair, dressed in a blue cloak. She's holding a staff in one of her hands. She is the Norse goddess Saga, the one who sees into the future. She is very wise. Saga is holding a golden cup in her hand, and she invites you to drink from it. It contains the elixir of inspiration, visions, dreams, and the magic of who you truly are. Feel how you drink from her golden cup and, as you do, you realize you are drinking directly from the Goddess of Magic.

Saga explains that you have the power within you to weave a new story for your life, and that it is you who chooses the threads you weave with. These threads are filled with the energy you choose to infuse your thoughts, words, and actions with.

Weave a new story into being

She asks you to take a moment to notice what you want to weave into your life—the new story you want to weave into being. Notice the energy you want to fill this story with.

Feel, see, hear, and notice how you start to spin and weave your light, wisdom, magic, love, and fierce compassion into this new story you are birthing into the world, through the threads you choose to weave with.

Weave in your soul gifts, feminine power, visions, dreams, prayers, and intentions.

Weave in beautiful golden threads, filled with the glowing healing light from the sun, and silvery threads, filled with the intuitive soft light from the moon.

Weave in the magic of starlight that shimmers so beautifully in the darkness of the night, the sacredness of the ancient forests, the freedom of the vast oceans, the wisdom of the old mountains, and the miracle of the early morning rays of the sun, that bring the promise of a new day.

Weave in all the beauty, magic, and sacredness of life into the new story for the future.

Your new mythic map

Know deep within your heart and soul that this is the magical power you have awakened within you; the power to choose to weave all these visions, dreams, and wisdom into a new mythic map, a map that is now filled with all the positive resources, soul gifts, and feminine magic you have received as you've moved through this sacred journey.

It is this new mythic map you are now weaving into being, where you are being the Wise Woman, seeing through the spiritual eye of your heart, sharing your healing medicine and beautiful light with the world.

Then say goodbye to Saga, the Valkyries, and the norns.

And now it is time for you to journey back, so feel how you come back to the Tree of Life.

Becoming the Tree of Life

Step inside it, bringing your staff with you.

Feel your roots going deep down into the sacred darkness, and your branches reaching high up into the magical light.

Feel the presence of the Dark Mother within you, in your roots, in your bones, and in your blood. Feel how she is holding you, loving you, healing you and nourishing you from within.

Feel the presence of the Light Mothers above you and all around you. Open up to receive their healing, golden rays of light, into you. Let yourself breathe in their healing light and medicine for you, filling your lungs with their magic, with their life force. Let it flow from your lungs and into your blood, filling your blood with their love for you.

Within your blood, you now have the medicine of the Dark Mothers and the Light Mothers, and for every heartbeat, this medicine flows through your body, nourishing and sustaining you.

You are held and loved and supported by the Divine Mothers of Darkness and Light, always and in all ways.

Thank them, and then tune into the light that shines in your mystical heart, the light that is a portal between the worlds.

Journey back through the portal

Take a deep breath in and, as you breathe out, feel how you journey through this portal now, coming back into your body, back into the here and now, bringing with you all your insights, learnings, wisdom, and gifts.

Take another deep breath in and, as you breathe out, feel how you share these insights, learnings, wisdom, and gifts with the world, in a way that helps and supports others, and you.

Take another deep breath in and, as you breathe out, you can open your eyes.

⌒

Take a moment now to write down your insights and learnings. Make sure that you write down the insights you've had on how you can use your time, energy, and focus with more wisdom.

Write down the soul gifts and healing medicine you are meant to share.

Write down the steps you are meant to take, this week, this month and for the next coming year. These steps will give you the structure you need for all of this to be born through you.

Write down the commitment you now want to make to your heart, a commitment that will help you to be the Wise Woman that you are.

Trust that, as you act on this new commitment, as you listen to your heart's loving wisdom guiding you to the inspired action you are meant to take, you weave the healing medicine from the Wise Woman into your life, into your community, and into the world.

You can start this letter with the words:

What my heart's loving wisdom wants me
to weave into my world is ...

The wisdom you write down now, from your heart, is the new *mythic* map you will take with you into your life. A new mythic map filled with all the soul gifts, healing medicine, feminine power, and ancient magic that you have awakened within you, where you are seeing through the eye of the heart, being the Wise Woman that you are.

Closing Words

You already have within you everything you need
to turn your dreams into reality.
—*Wallace D. Wattles*

Thank you for having taken this journey of healing, transformation, magic, and rebirth with me, during which you have dived deep into the medicine found in your mystical heart and awakened the Wise Woman within. You are now meant to share your heart's loving wisdom with those you meet, weaving your unique light and soul essence into your world.

You can revisit any chapters any time you need to connect more deeply with the frequency of that particular medicine.

To tune into your heart, in a gentle way, I recommend you listen to the shamanic journey into your heart (chapter one).

When you want to balance your nervous system, take the shamanic journey to heal and cleanse your chakras and tune into the Tree of Life (chapter two).

When you feel you have outgrown an old skin, listen to the shamanic journey to release the past and heal your ancestral lineage (chapter three).

Any time you need to transform and heal deeply, take the shamanic journey through the seven gates into the underworld (chapter four).

When you want to receive divine inspiration and light-filled new dreams, listen to the shamanic journey where you meet the Spirit Weavers (chapter five).

To receive more nourishment and light for your dreams to grow, listen to the shamanic journey to ignite your inner magic (chapter six).

When it is time for you to emerge, renewed, listen to the shamanic journey of initiation and rebirth (chapter seven).

For those times when you want to awaken the eye in your heart and be initiated into your feminine magic and creative power, do the shamanic journey with Mary Magdalene (chapter eight).

And when you want to focus on turning your heart's dreams into reality, take our final shamanic journey where you fly with the *Valkyries* using your time, energy, and focus wisely, so that you can weave your heart's wisdom and loving dreams into your life (chapter nine).

Each time you do one of these shamanic journeys, you'll awaken another layer of feminine wisdom and magic within you, so it is highly beneficial to do these journeys several times. I do them regularly myself.

I will now finish our healing journey together with a final prayer to the Divine Mothers of Darkness and Light, a prayer you can tune into any time to connect with them more deeply.

Thank you so much for being on this journey with me. Sending you lots of love, from my heart to yours.

Much love, Cissi

Closing Prayer to the Divine Mothers of Darkness and Light

This surrendering prayer has been inspired by the teachings from the Dark Mothers and Light Mothers, and from *A Course in Miracles*—especially the healer's prayer.

You can access the recording of this prayer (9 minutes long) on cissiwilliams.com/heart.

Beautiful Divine Mothers of Darkness and Light,

Thank you for holding me and supporting me with your love—like a loving, ancient mother within my bones—flowing through my blood, sustaining me from within my core.

Thank you for strengthening my roots, and for guiding me on my journey into the sacred darkness, so I can discover the wisdom, and magic, and soul gifts I came here to share with the world.

Thank you for filling me with new inspiration and life force for every breath I take, and for nourishing me with your magical light from the heavens, so I can grow, expand, and blossom, into an expression of your love, an embodiment of your wisdom—so I can be the Wise woman you know I am.

I now know, deep within my bones, that I'm here only to be truly helpful, and to represent You, Ancient Divine Mothers of Darkness and Light, who sent me.

I don't have to worry about what to say or what to do, because I know, YOU will direct me.

And I'm content to be wherever you want me to be, knowing you will go there with me.

And I trust that I will be healed, as I let you teach me how to heal.

So Dear Divine Mothers of Darkness and Light I give my path to you

May you be in charge because I will follow you

Certain that your direction gives me peace

So, show me where to go, what to do

What to say and to whom

I am ready to follow your lead.

And then, be in stillness, whilst repeating this question silently in your mind to the Divine Mothers of Darkness and Light:

How may I serve you?

Just be still and allow yourself to receive the answer. It may come as a feeling, an inner knowing, a vision, or you may hear their answer. But trust that they will answer you. Let their answer be revealed to you, from within the stillness.

How may I serve you?

Beautiful Divine Mothers of Darkness and Light.

I am ready to be an embodiment of your loving wisdom.

I am ready to speak your truth and be an expression of your light and feminine magic.

I'm ready to BE the Wise Woman that I am.

And so it is. And so it is. And so it is.

Blessed be. Blessed be. Blessed be.

Resources

Suggested Reading

The Seed of Yggdrasil by Maria Kvilhaug

The Gospel of the Beloved Companion by Jehanne de Quillan

The Gospel of Mary of Magdala by Karen L. King

The Meaning of Mary Magdalene by Cynthia Bourgeault

Mary Magdalene Revealed by Meggan Watterson

Women who Run with the Wolves by Clarissa Pinkola Estés

The Great Cosmic Mother: Rediscovering the Religion of the Earth by Monica Sjöö and Barbara Mor

Warrior Goddess Training: Become the Woman You Are Meant to Be by HeatherAsh Amara

Wild, Willing, and Wise by HeatherAsh Amara

Womb Awakening: Initiatory Wisdom from the Creatrix of All Life by Seren and Azra Bertrand

Magdalene Mysteries: The Left-Hand Path of the Feminine Christ by Seren and Azra Bertrand

You are a Goddess: Working with the Sacred Feminine to Awaken, Heal and Transform by Sophie Bashford

Cerridwen: Celtic Goddess of Inspiration by Kristoffer Hughes

Goddesses: Mysteries of the Feminine Divine by Joseph Campbell

Witches and Pagans: Women in European Folk Religion, 700-1100 by Max Dashu

Dancing in the Flames: The Dark Goddess in the Transformation of Consciousness by Marion Woodman, Elinor Dickson

Witchcraze: New History of the European Witch Hunts by Anne Llewellyn Barstow

The Modern Witchcraft Guide to the Wheel of the Year: From Samhain to Yule, Your Guide to the Wiccan Holidays (Modern Witchcraft Magic, Spells, Rituals) by Judy Ann Nock

Soul Retrieval: Mending the Fragmented Self by Sandra Ingerman

Energy Strands: The Ultimate Guide to Clearing the Cords That Are Constricting Your Life by Denise Linn

Kindling the Native Spirit: Sacred Practices for Everyday Life by Denise Linn

Rise Sister Rise: A Guide to Unleashing the Wise, Wild Woman Within by Rebecca Campbell

You Are the Medicine: 13 Moons of Indigenous Wisdom, Ancestral Connection, and Animal Spirit Guidance by Asha Frost

Spells for Living Well: A Witch's Guide for Manifesting Change, Well-being, and Wonder by Phyllis Curott

Descent & Rising: Women's Stories & the Embodiment of the Inanna Myth by Carly Mountain

Burning Woman by Lucy H. Pearce

A Fierce Heart: Finding Strength, Wisdom, and Courage in Any Moment by Spring Washam

Drawing Down the Moon: Witches, Druids, Goddess-Worshippers, and Other Pagans in America by Margot Adler

Aspecting the Goddess: Drawing Down the Divine Feminine by Jane Meredith

The Spiral Dance: A Rebirth of the Ancient Religion of the Great Goddess by Starhawk

Priestess of Avalon, Priestess of the Goddess: A Renewed Spiritual Path for the 21st Century by Kathy Jones

Love is the Answer: Creating Positive Relationships by Gerald Jampolsky and Diane Cirincione

The Path of She: Book of Sabbats by Karen Clark

A Course in Miracles by Foundation for Inner Peace

A Return to Love by Marianne Williamson

Illuminata by Marianne Williamson

Oracle decks that help you tune into Nature's Wisdom & the Divine Feminine

The Mystique of Mary Magdalene: An Oracle of Love by
    Cheryl Yambrach Rose

The Mary Magdalene Oracle by Meggan Watterson

The Divine Feminine Oracle by Meggan Watterson

Goddesses, Gods and Guardians Oracle Cards by Sophie Bashford

The Sacred Medicine Oracle by Asha Frost

Goddess Power Oracle by Colette Baron-Reid

Mystical Shaman Oracle by Alberto Villoldo, Colette Baron-Reid,
    Marcela Lobos

The Sacred Forest Oracle by Denise Linn

The Rose Oracle by Rebecca Campbell

The Ancient Stones Oracle by Rebecca Campbell

The Witches' Wisdom Tarot by Phyllis Curott

Witches' Wisdom Oracle by Barbara Meiklejohn-Free and
    Flavia Kate Peters

Moonology™ *Oracle* by Yasmin Boland

Suggested guided shamanic journeys and meditations to listen to

Shamanic journeys and meditations on *Awaken Your Inner Wisdom*
    podcast

Journeys into Past Lives with Denise Linn

33 Spirit Journeys with Denise Linn

Shamanic Visioning with Sandra Ingerman

The Soul Retrieval Journey: Seeing in the Dark with Sandra Ingerman

Guided shamanic journeys with HeatherAsh Amara

Guided shamanic journeys with Linda Fitch

Guided shamanic journeys with Jane Burns

Guided shamanic journeys with Seren Bertrand

Guided shamanic womb journeys with Deborah Stanley

Guided meditations with Asha Frost

Guided meditations with Sophie Bashford

Guided meditations with Rebecca Campbell

Guided meditations with Colette Baron-Reid

Guided meditations with Alana Fairchild

Guided meditations with Elayne Kalila

Guided meditations with Meggan Watterson

Guided meditations with Chameli Ardagh

Websites with more inspiration

cissiwilliams.com

nordiclight.academy

innerwisdom.courses

warriorgoddess.com

heatherashamara.com

goddesstemple.co.uk

bladehoner.wordpress.com

azrabertrand.com

serenbertrand.com

ashafrost.com

sophiebashford.com

phylliscurott.com

deniselinnseminars.com

sandraingerman.com

rebeccacampbell.me

colettebaronreid.com

awakeningwomen.com

elaynekalila.com

lookwithininstitute.com

megganwatterson.com

lindalfitch.com

michellemacewan.com.au

journeystothesoul.com

theshiftnetwork.com

Shamanic Journeys
and Exercises

Acknowledgements

Thank you to my parents, who gave me life and provided me with the contrast I needed to embark on my healing journey. I love you deeply and will always carry you in my heart.

Thank you to my husband, who always has my back, no matter how deep I descend into the darkness of the cauldron or how high I fly into the light. I know you are always there, like a constant beacon of light and strength. You are my rock, my anchor, my best friend, my soul mate, and I love you more than words can express. Meeting you opened the door to a life filled with love and happiness.

Thank you to my two beautiful daughters, who are like radiant stars, each shining in their own unique way. Being your mum is the greatest blessing of my life, and seeing you spread your wings and fly into the world fills my heart with immense joy.

Thank you to my shamanic sister Debbie Price. You mean more to me than you'll ever know, and your friendship is a blessing from the Divine Mother. And thank you to my shamanic sister Lindsey Marquez. I'm so grateful for you being with us in the cauldron—our very own Dragon Mother! I love how we are like three shamanic witch-priestesses, journeying into the World of Spirit to bring through this ancient medicine. Meeting up with you regularly in Glastonbury to dive deep into the magic of Seidr is such a gift!

Thank you to all my sisters—together, we are bringing each other back home to the truth of who we are, awakening this deep feminine magic found in our ancestral lineages.

A special thank you to Sabine Weeke, from Findhorn Press and Inner Traditions, who has been the spiritual midwife helping to birth this book into the world. I'm forever grateful for your support, kindness, and encouragement.

Thank you to Elaine O'Neill for her invaluable developmental editing input, and to Susan Kemp and Jaime Fleres for their magical spirit-weaver editing skills. You are amazing!

Thank you to HeatherAsh Amara, who graciously agreed to write the foreword for this book. I always cherish our chats, and you were one of the first people I spoke with after my mum's passing. Your compassion was like a soothing balm that helped heal my grief-stricken heart.

Thank you to all the amazing trailblazers who have gone before me and illuminated the path. You have forever changed me—through your books, oracle decks, guided shamanic journeys, and the wisdom you share. One of the greatest gifts of the podcast is that I've been able to connect with you in person!! Amazing! There are so many of you who have profoundly impacted me, many who have kindly written endorsements for this book. I'm deeply grateful for the light you shine into our world.

A special thank you to Norse scholar Maria Kvilhaug for her incredible research on the Norse Sagas, and to Meggan Watterson, Karen King, Jehanne de Quillan, and Cynthia Bourgeault for their research on Mary Magdalene. Deep gratitude to Azra and Seren Bertrand for their amazing research found in the books *Womb Awakening* and *Magdalene Mysteries*, as well as their teachings on Feminine Magic and Biomancy through their online courses.

I also want to thank Chameli Ardagh for her beautiful gift in decoding goddess myths, as well as Elayne Kalila, Zindra Andersson, Andrew Harvey, Clarissa Pinkola Estés, and the Glastonbury Goddess Temple, for sharing the teachings of the sacred feminine in such a multifaceted way. Additionally, my gratitude extends to all my shamanic teachers for opening the door into the World of Spirit, and to the amazing Denise Linn, who helped me heal deeply, thanks to her shamanic journeys and guided meditations, already back in the early 90s.

Deep appreciation to my heart and my body, who helped me remember this ancient wisdom that was wired into my DNA, flowing through my veins, and embedded within my bones. Thank you for helping me awaken!

And finally, deep gratitude to the Divine Mothers of Darkness and Light, who are my spiritual teachers, guides, and mentors. You have forever altered me.

With deep love and gratitude,

Cissi Williams

About the Author

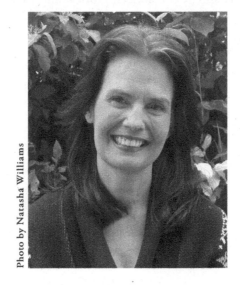

Photo by Natasha Williams

Cissi Williams is an osteopath, naturopath, shamanic practitioner, NLP trainer, master practitioner in hypnosis, and a teacher of energy medicine, mysticism, shamanic healing, and Seidr. She's initiated as a Priestess of Freya, Tradition Keeper of the Völva (Seidr and Norse shamanism and magic).

She started her healing journey in 1992, when she had her first dark night of the soul experience. This brought her into an immense darkness, where she finally fell on her knees and prayed. Her prayer was answered in the form of three books: *The Power Is Within You* by Louise Hay, *Love Is the Answer* by Gerald Jampolsky, and *Creative Visualization* by Shakti Gawain. As she read these books, she could feel the darkness lift, and through doing the exercises outlined in the books, she healed her depression in six weeks. She then knew that we have the power to heal within us.

This led her to want to learn more about health and healing, so she earned a four-year university degree in London (she qualified in 1997 with First Class Honours in Osteopathic Medicine). She worked for many years in private practice at an orthopaedic clinic and at a doctor's surgery, where she specialized in paediatric and cranial osteopathy.

In 2002, she started her training in NLP and hypnosis, which later led her into the world of shamanism, and she's undertaken shamanic training from various wisdom traditions, including Norse, Celtic, and Incan.

Cissi has developed a unique way of working with shamanic energy medicine based on her grounded understanding of the body (through her work as an osteopath and naturopath); the mind (through her work in NLP and hypnosis); the soul (through shamanic and mystical traditions); and spirit (through *A Course in Miracles*, mysticism, and shamanic journeying).

Cissi runs trainings in shamanic energy medicine and Seidr Magic, through Nordic Light Academy of Energy Medicine, training students to become certified practitioners and master practitioners in shamanic energy medicine, and Shamanic Priestesses & Tradition Keepers of the Völva, the Path of the Wise Woman in Norse Shamanism and Seidr Magic.

Her work has been featured on *The Shift Network* and in various magazines, such as *Kindred Spirit, Hälsa, Nära, Mind, Body & Spirit, Inspire*, and *Inspired Wellbeing*, as well as on online summits such as the Shamanic Wisdom Summit, Wise Women Summit, Shamanic Dreamkeepers Summit, Witches Summit, SheHEALS Summit, and her own yearly Winter Solstice Summit.

Cissi is originally from Sweden. Her maternal ancestry traces back to the far north of Sweden, Lapland, and Finland. Her maternal bloodline, specifically the maternal haplogroup inherited from mother to daughter, is common among the Sami community—the nomadic people of northern Scandinavia.

Her ancestry on her father's side goes all the way back to the Vikings through her paternal grandmother, where it enters the Scandinavian royal bloodline in the 1200s. This lineage includes Queen Ingeborg Eriksdotter of Sweden, King Eric X of Sweden, the Viking King Valdemar the Great of Denmark, King Erik the Good of Denmark, and many others within the royal courts. Through her paternal grandfather, her bloodline traces back to the Walloons, descendants of the Celts.

She now lives with her husband and two daughters in a little village in the Cotswolds, Oxfordshire, England, UK.

To find out more visit **cissiwilliams.com** and **nordiclight.academy**.

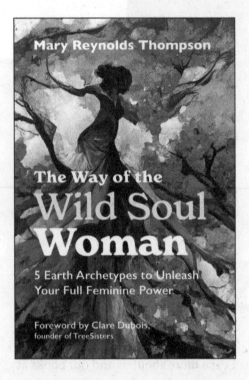

The Way of the Wild Soul Woman

by Mary Reynolds Thompson

ARE YOU READY TO REWILD YOUR SOUL and become a force of nature? Taking you on a journey of transformation and rebirth, Mary Reynolds Thompson reveals how to unleash your full feminine power and discover authenticity, creativity, and healing through initiation with ancient Earth Archetypes. Find rituals, exercises, and meditations to help you integrate each initiatory stage and embody the ways of a Wild Soul Woman.

979-8-88850-033-0